AORN

theclinics.com

PERIOPERATIVE NURSING CLINICS

Perioperative Environment 20/20 in 2020

George F. Nussbaum, PhD, RN, CNOR
Guest Editor

Patricia C. Seifert, RN, MSN, CNOR, CRNFA, FAAN
Consulting Editor

March 2008 • Volume 3 • Number 1

SAUNDERS

An Imprint of Elsevier, Inc.
PHILADELPHIA   LONDON   TORONTO   MONTREAL   SYDNEY   TOKYO

W.B. SAUNDERS COMPANY
A Division of Elsevier Inc.

Elsevier Inc. • 1600 John F. Kennedy Boulevard • Suite 1800 • Philadelphia, Pennsylvania 19103-2899

http://www.periopnursing.theclinics.com

PERIOPERATIVE NURSING CLINICS
March 2008
Editor: Alexandra Gavenda

Volume 3, Number 1
ISSN 1556-7931
ISBN-13: 978-1-4160-5778-9
ISBN-10: 1-4160-5778-1

Perioperative Nursing Clinics (ISSN 1556-7931) is published quarterly by Elsevier, 360 Park Avenue South, New York, NY 10010. Months of issue are March, June, September and December. Business and Editorial Office: 1600 John F. Kennedy Blvd., Ste. 1800, Philadelphia, PA 19103-2899. Accounting and Circulation Offices: 6277 Sea Harbor Dr, Orlando, FL 32887-4800. Periodicals postage paid at New York, NY and at additional mailing offices.

POSTMASTER: Send change of address to *Perioperative Nursing Clinics,* Elsevier, Periodicals Department, 6277 Sea Harbor Dr, Orlando, FL 32887-4800. Customer Service: 1-800-654-2452 (US). From outside the United States, call 1-407-563-6020. Fax: 1-407-363-9661. E-mail: JournalsCustomer Service-usa@elsevier.com.

Printed in the United States of America.

CONSULTING EDITOR

PATRICIA C. SEIFERT, RN, MSN, CNOR, CRNFA, FAAN, Education Coordinator, Cardiovascular Operating Room, Inova Heart and Vascular Institute, Falls Church, Virginia

GUEST EDITOR

GEORGE F. NUSSBAUM, PhD, RN, CNOR, Clinical Planner, Halff Associates; Architecture and Engineering, Inc., Dallas, Texas; Assistant Professor, Graduate School of Nursing, Perioperative Clinical Nurse Specialist Program, Uniformed Services University, Bethesda, Maryland

CONTRIBUTORS

SANDRA C. BIBB, DNSc, RN, Associate Professor of Nursing, and Chair, Department of Health Systems, Risk, and Contingency Management; Research Director, Perioperative Clinical Nurse Specialist Program, Graduate School of Nursing, Uniformed Services University of the Health Sciences, Bethesda, Maryland

CHIP DAVIS, BA, Composer, Mannheim Steamroller, Omaha, Nebraska

KAREN D. DUNLAP, MSN, RN, CNOR, Lieutenant Colonel, Army Nurse Corps; Chief, Nursing Performance Improvement, Walter Reed Army Medical Center, Washington, DC

MARY S. HULL, LTC, AN, RN, MS, PMH-NP, Nurse Manager, Department of Nursing, Inpatient Psychiatry, Landstuhl Regional Medical Center; Officer in Charge, Fitness Team, 254th Combat Stress Control Detachment, Miesau, Germany

ERIN LAWLER, MS, Human Factors Engineer, Department of Defense Patient Safety Center, Silver Spring, Maryland

SUSAN M. MYERS, RN, MSN, Healthcare Planner, The Innova Group, Georgetown, Texas

GEORGE F. NUSSBAUM, PhD, RN, CNOR, Clinical Planner, Halff Associates; Architecture and Engineering, Inc., Dallas, Texas; Assistant Professor, Graduate School of Nursing, Perioperative Clinical Nurse Specialist Program, Uniformed Services University, Bethesda, Maryland

A. RAY PENTECOST III, DrPH, AIA, ACHA, Vice President and Director of Healthcare Architecture, Clark Nexsen, Norfolk, Virginia

KEVIN SCHLAHT, AIA, MArch, MBA, President, The Innova Group, Georgetown, Texas

CHARLOTTE M. SHELL, MSN, RN, Major, Army Nurse Corps; Quality Improvement Nurse, Nursing Services, Brooke Army Medical Center, Fort Sam, Houston, Texas

RANDY TOMASZEWSKI, RN, BSN, MBA, Vice President of Marketing, Skytron, Grand Rapids, Michigan

ELIZABETH A.P. VANE, LTC, AN, RN, MS, CNOR, Chief, Department of Nursing, Perioperative Nursing Services, Landstuhl Regional Medical Center, Germany

LINDA J. WANZER, MSN, RN, CNOR, COL, AN, Assistant Professor of Nursing, and Director, Perioperative Clinical Nurse Specialist Program, Graduate School of Nursing, Uniformed Services University of the Health Sciences, Bethesda, Maryland

CONTENTS

> The foundation for evidence-based decision making has been established in the perioperative environment, but the ongoing challenge for perioperative nurses is to validate, modify, or develop practice guidelines that support evidence-based practice. To accomplish these tasks successfully, perioperative nurses must be well versed in the research and literature review processes and must understand the underlying principles of rigor and replicability when determining the evidence using published literature. The purpose of this article is to outline an identifying, organizing, and synthesizing strategy for determining the evidence, using the integrative research review and a standard set of research process tools designed to address issues related to rigor and replication.

> The foundation of patient safety was started by Florence Nightingale in 1854 and was enhanced in 1910 by Dr. Ernest Codman and his "end result system of standardization." In 1951, the Joint Commission on Accreditation of Hospitals (now the Joint Commission) was established. The decades since then have seen further enhancements in the scope of the commission's activities and an increase in the number of organizations under its wings. During the twenty-first century, the Joint Commission has continued to evolve, with the establishment of the sentinel event policy and the development of a standards improvement initiative. Only with continued outcomes management and evidence-based medicine will health care continue to move toward improved patient safety and optimal patient care.

> Nursing is a high-risk occupation for work-related musculoskeletal disorders, usually caused by the strain of lifting and moving patients. These injuries are financially costly to

health care organizations and increase significantly the workforce necessary to deliver health care effectively, efficiently, and safely. Opportunities to integrate innovative and safe patient-handling technologies abound. As the patient safety movement evolves, more evidence-based research is needed with respect to design interventions that minimize patient handling. One possible solution is to use multifunctional beds to reduce musculoskeletal disorders among caregivers.

Musculoskeletal injuries among nursing personnel required to lift and laterally transfer patients manually carries substantial injury, salary, and personnel replacement costs per incident. Unintended hypothermia in surgical patients has been researched and published with resulting recommendations, yet the problem remains. The primary purpose of this article is to question the potential effects that the use of a single transport-procedure-recovery platform might provide. The full range of surgical care that can be delivered using these platforms has not been explored, in part because of the newness of the concept. Numerous potential advantages will not be realized if a specific platform is not able to perform as well as, or better than, the current standard operating room tables and allow the performance of most of the procedures currently being performed.

Whether your operating room design project involves renovation, new construction, or a little of both, operating room equipment layout planning and implementation strategies can be challenging, with available technologies representing a staggering array of options. Having a clear understanding of your own facility's future goals is a big step toward arriving at the best solution to meet your facility's growth needs. The most successful plan involves a team effort and multidisciplinary input from key clinical end users and support personnel. The goal should always be maximum flexibility and adaptability to anticipated future needs.

Facility planning for perioperative services is no longer limited to clinical areas directly in support of operating room surgical cases. For example, the advent of interventional procedures requiring various levels of conscious sedation and anesthesia in specialties such as gastroenterology, radiology, and urology impact support areas such as preadmissions, preoperative processing, and the postanesthesia care unit. Additionally, the health care facility venue in which perioperative services is provided impacts facility planning for these same support areas. This article explores required health care facility planning for perioperative services before the development of the facility design to ensure all users of perioperative support spaces are planned for adequately.

The health care industry and, more specifically, the perioperative setting have a 30-year history of acquiring a complete disposable habit. The fast-paced nature of perioperative nursing allows little time to contemplate the costs or impact of these practices; however, nurses are increasingly aware and concerned for their own safety and the safety of those who may be exposed to potential disease-causing materials. It seems to be the time to reconsider the benefits and liabilities of our practice habits. In the absence of definitive, conclusive, and compelling unbiased scientific evidence, we are directed by industry rather than by our own profession.

FORTHCOMING ISSUES

RECENT ISSUES

ELSEVIER
SAUNDERS

Perioperative Nursing Clinics 3 (2008) ix–x

PERIOPERATIVE
NURSING
CLINICS

Foreword

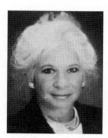

Patricia C. Seifert, RN, MSN, CNOR,
CRNFA, FAAN
Consulting Editor

Planning for the future always starts in the past—a notion that became readily apparent in December 2007 when I visited Egypt, a country that, in ancient times, focused on meticulous future planning. The ancient Egyptians set a standard by ensuring an adequate supply of food, physical and spiritual comfort, and protection from injury in the next life. Five thousand years later, the idea of future planning continues to rely on understanding the past, evaluating current resources, and projecting future needs and capabilities.

This issue of *Perioperative Nursing Clinics* looks at a variety of topics that address the future of surgical care in a manner that integrates past, present, and future considerations. Guest Editor Dr. George Nussbaum has selected and coordinated articles that address the major themes of patient and staff safety, research and evidence-based practice, ergonomically sensitive facility planning, waste management, and the future impact on surgery being driven by decoding of the genome and refinement of imaging and other technologies. Readers will appreciate the importance, and the necessity, of focusing on mundane concepts (eg, "waste management") and more sublime visions (eg, "ambient nature sounds" and three-dimensional "virtual" procedures) that collectively reflect the multiple facets of health care.

Many of the articles refer to historical precedents when describing future trends. Shell and Dunlap refer to Florence Nightingale and Dr Ernest Codman—two icons of nursing and surgery, respectively—when discussing future quality initiatives to enhance patient safety. The authors stress the importance of moving beyond measurement to achieve a healthcare system that stresses accountability for preventable errors. Vane and Hull address the issue of staff safety in the context of promoting resiliency and mental fitness among perioperative team members during times of war and natural disasters.

Nussbaum addresses a more common, but nonetheless critical daily occurrence in operating rooms (ORs) (moving patients), and he illustrates the significant potential injuries associated with this routine act: staff musculoskeletal injuries, patient hypothermia, and increased risk for infection. Nussbaum demonstrates clinical, operational, and financial advantages to using a single vehicle for transport and treatment in selected patient populations. Staff safety is promoted further in Lawler's article that discusses not only patient transfers, but also the extensive movement of surgical equipment and supplies, prolonged standing, and awkward positions; the author discusses newer design interventions that can minimize injury and promote safety. Tomaszewski

doi:10.1016/j.cpen.2008.01.001

provides an overview of OR suite designs of the future that incorporate not only safety features, but also communication systems, 3-dimensional imaging capabilities, data management, and information repositories. The OR of the future will be adaptable, flexible, and user-friendly while "keeping it simple." Myers and Schlaht look at perioperative functions in the pre-, intra- and postoperative setting and offer practical "voice-of-experience" recommendations for design features that can facilitate newer surgical technologies and operative trends.

Future ORs will become centers of evidence-based practice. Bibb and Wanzer offer in-depth research process tools for identifying, organizing, and synthesizing evidence for decision-making. Future ORs also will incorporate more aesthetic components. Davis and Nussbaum write about using nature sounds and music to reduce anxiety, stress, and pain for patients and staff. The ancient Romans and Greeks believed in the power of music to heal. More current research has confirmed the value of music and serves as the conceptual underpinning for incorporating stress-reducing ambient sound into future designs.

Although music can "soothe the savage breast," hospital waste does not have the same charm. However, the topic of "trash" cannot be omitted from any discussion of the future. Nussbaum has taken an unexciting topic and turned it into an article that is eye-opening and critically

important not only for patients and staff, but also for the greater community. Few subjects stir as much controversy as the disposal of waste. The impact on the environment and the cost considerations make this an important topic.

Finally, Pentecost, Bardwell and Bonine look at the implications for future healthcare design from an architect's perspective. The authors suggest short- and long-term research issues (such as a "robotic juke box circulating nurse") and emphasize the importance of evidence-based design. Their predictions of the types of surgery that will be performed and the tools and technologies that will be employed make fascinating reading.

This issue is a rich blend of the practical and the ideal. When we consider what will be, it is appropriate that we look at what we want and how best to make it work. Dr. Nussbaum and his authors have provided readers with an abundant supply of both.

Patricia C. Seifert, RN, MSN, CNOR, CRNFA, FAAN
Cardiovascular Operating Room
Inova Heart and Vascular Institute
3300 Gallows Road
Falls Church, VA 22042, USA

E-mail address: patricia.seifert@inova.org

PERIOPERATIVE
NURSING
CLINICS

Perioperative Nursing Clinics 3 (2008) xi–xii

Preface

The notion of an "operating room of the future" is an intriguing concept. As a university professor in a perioperative graduate program, I frequently assign students the task of discovering the meanings and predictions of this phenomenon. This academic exercise most often yields very little substantive results. To most of us, the "operating room of the future" creates a mental picture of high technology equipment, robotics, and advanced telecommunication strategies. Equipment vendors capitalize on the term and create an array of ceiling-mounted booms, wall-mounted monitors displaying patient information, and control consoles to support the advancing technologies.

Early this year I discovered the "operating room of the future" is a government-funded applied research project conducted at the Massachusetts General Hospital in Boston, Massachusetts that is intended to solve process issues. The study resulted in numerous publications illustrating parallel process activities that improve patient flow, recovery room availability, and room turnover times. I had the distinct opportunity to visit the research teams at the Massachusetts General Hospital and to witness firsthand the origin of the initial "operating room of the future."

Intrigued by the predictive nature of the environment in which the practice of operating room nursing is evolving, Patricia Seifert and I collaborated to produce the informative content for this issue of Perioperative Nursing Clinics. I offer my sincere appreciation to Patricia as the consulting editor for her support, encouragement, and guidance in the creation of the final product.

The immediate goal for this publication was to cast a wide global net that conceivably would create a 20/20 vision of the perioperative future. The results presented in this edition of the Perioperative Nursing Clinics come from professionals engaged in a wide and diverse range of disciplines including academia, The Joint Commission, industry, patient and staff safety, architectural master planners, medical futurists, music therapy composers, perioperative clinicians, clinical planners, and researchers. The fundamental principle for all of the content presented is grounded in the assumption that validated research provides the foundation upon which decisions regarding operating room and sterile processing department renovation or new designs of future facilities are established. A tremendous standardization tool is included in this issue that evaluates the evidence in published literature reviews. Researchers and futurists propose how the delivery of surgical healthcare may be delivered and projected based upon genetic factors that predict expected surgical requirements for individuals. Several articles address staff and patient safety with respect to patient transport, hypothermia, lateral transfers, staff injury, and alternative methods in the management of perioperative waste.

In an effort to capture the 20/20 vision of perioperative nursing, I included the efforts conducted in Landstuhl, Germany to support the staff members providing perioperative care for our nation's wounded warriors. Globally, and with increasing frequency, perioperative nurses are called to provide care and support for medically related military and civilian disasters and mass traumatic injuries. As perioperative professionals, we need to better understand the issues associated with staff compassion fatigue and resiliency strategies required in providing care for the health care givers.

The underlying premise presented by the authors in this issue is to offer solutions to the growing concerns that we face now and will continue to face as troubling issues occur in the near future. The authors deliberately highlight the current and future research that is needed to establish valid evidence upon which future design, staffing, and support elements are created on our way to the year 2020.

George F. Nussbaum, PhD, RN, CNOR
Graduate School of Nursing
Perioperative Clinical Nurse Specialist Program
Uniformed Services University
4301 Jones Bridge Road
Bethesda, MD 20814, USA

E-mail address: nussbaumgf@verizon.net

ELSEVIER
SAUNDERS

PERIOPERATIVE
NURSING
CLINICS

Perioperative Nursing Clinics 3 (2008) 1–17

Determining the Evidence in the Perioperative Environment: Standardizing Research Process Tools for Conducting the Integrative Literature Review

Sandra C. Bibb, DNSc, RN*,
Linda J. Wanzer, MSN, RN, CNOR, COL, AN

Graduate School of Nursing, Uniformed Services University of the Health Sciences, 4301 Jones Bridge Road, Bethesda, MD 20814-5119, USA

Evidenced-based practice is the integration of best research evidence with clinical expertise and client ideals in the delivery of quality health care [1]. Within the discipline of nursing, evidence-based practice "refers to nursing practice that uses research findings as the foundation for nurses' decisions, activities, and interactions with clients" [2]. Evidence-based practice requires ongoing conduction of studies and synthesis of published literature to address relevant practice problems [3–6]. Hence, knowledge of the research process, capability in application of standards for rigor ("use of discipline, scrupulous adherence to detail, and strict accuracy" [3]), and replicability ("reproducing or repeating a study to determine whether similar findings will be obtained" [3]) when synthesizing the published literature, are fundamental to determining the evidence for practice.

The purpose of this article is to outline an identifying, organizing, and synthesizing (IOS) strategy designed to standardize the process tools used when conducting the integrative literature review. The goal of the IOS strategy is to promote research and evidence-based practice in advanced practice nursing and to address issues related to

rigor and replication in synthesizing published literature by standardizing the use of a specific set of process tools. The IOS strategy was developed for use by perioperative advanced practice nursing students, but application and use of these process tools is applicable across all specialties and advanced practice nursing clinical settings.

Literature reviews and evidence-based practice

A literature review "is an organized written presentation of what has been published on a topic by scholars" [3]. Most often, this broad definition of literature review refers to introductions to primary research study protocols or written reports that are not generally constructed following standard principles for rigor and replicability. In contrast, a literature review conducted as secondary research is based on a clearly constructed research question and is guided by explicit methods to identify, organize, and synthesize relevant literature, often for the purpose of contributing to evidence-based practice [7–11].

The mounting emphasis on evidence-based practice emphasizes the value of the literature review conducted as secondary research [7–9, 11,12]. These types of research reviews are held to high standards of rigor and replicability and are commonly classified in the nursing literature as integrative, systematic, meta-analysis, or meta-synthesis (see Refs. [3–6,10,11,13–16]). An integrative literature review is a summary and analysis of previous empiric or theoretic literature to provide

The views expressed are those of the authors and do not reflect the official policy or position of the Uniformed Services University of the Health Sciences, the Department of the Defense, or the United States government.

* Corresponding author.

E-mail address: sbibb@usuhs.mil (S.C. Bibb).

a broader understanding of a phenomenon of interest [3,7,11,17]. The scope of the integrative review can be narrow or broad, and the type of analysis is narrative. A systematic review is "a rigorous and systematic literature search, using a well-defined question, and strict criteria for study inclusion and evaluation" [4]. The scope of the systematic review is narrow and the type of analysis can be narrative or statistical [8,17]. Meta-analyses are often found in systematic reviews and are the statistical reanalysis of data from studies with similar hypotheses to calculate the overall effect, the magnitude of effect, and subsample effects [4,7,17,18]. The scope for meta-analyses is narrow and the type of analysis is statistical. Meta-synthesis, the summary and analysis of qualitative research, is "the theories, grand narratives, generalizations, or interpretive translations produced from the integration or comparison of findings from qualitative studies" [6].

"Traditional evidence hierarchies were developed specifically to address questions of efficacy and effectiveness and involved assessing research according to study design with the randomized trial as the premier form of evidence" [15]. Conventionally, determining the evidence within these well-established hierarchies has focused primarily on systematic reviews and meta-analyses. However, recent growth in, and emphasis on, evidence-based practice has increased the requirement for all types of literature reviews, and has intensified the concentration on standards for rigor and replicability for each type of secondary research review (integrative, systematic, meta-analysis, or meta-synthesis) [7,11,13–17,19]. The integrative review provides for the inclusion of experimental and nonexperimental research and theoretic literature, and has the potential to play a greater role in evidence-based practice for nursing [11,15–17]. Therefore, the integrative research review was selected as the focus for development of the IOS strategy, and is the type of secondary research review presented in this article.

Evidence-based practice in the perioperative environment

The philosophy of evidence to guide practice decisions emerged in health care in the early 1970s, was operationalized as evidence-based medicine in the mid-1980s, and was introduced to perioperative nursing in the late 1990s [20–23]. Over the last 10 years, the emphasis on evidence as a foundation for practice decisions has gained momentum, and evidence-based practice has become the approach to introducing change in the clinical setting [15,24–26]. In addition, evidence-based practice decisions have become an important goal of health care providers, and an implicit expectation of health care organizations, insurers, and patients [21,27]. The evidence-based philosophy has evolved into a worldwide movement, challenging perioperative nursing to focus on research as a means of informing practice, and to analyze critically the delivery of care within the perioperative clinical environment [20,23,28]. To be effective in today's environment, perioperative advanced practice nurses must be clinically and technically competent; demonstrate independent judgment and skilled decision making; and promote positive outcomes through integration of clinical practice, education, managerial leadership, and research [27,29–31]. Thus, the challenge for today's perioperative nurse is to validate, modify, or develop practice guidelines that support the efficacy of the care delivered within the complex perioperative clinical environment [20,28,29]. To accomplish these tasks successfully, perioperative nurses must be well versed in the research and literature review processes, and must understand the underlying principles of rigor and replicability when determining the evidence using published literature.

The foundation for evidence-based practice has been established in the perioperative environment. In 2000, the Association of periOperative Registered Nurses (AORN) reviewed and, as appropriate, modified all published AORN guidelines and recommended practices to ensure that these documents were based on research or predicated by theoretic rationale and clinical expert opinion [20,22,32–34]. Yet, to sustain the momentum built by AORN, perioperative nurses will need to establish and maintain an active role in reviewing perioperative nursing practice and defining best practices, and must become involved in the process of discovery and validation [20,21,23,34]. The integrative literature review is a secondary research method that uses a uniform approach to identify, summarize, and analyze relevant literature. The integrative review process is closely aligned to the problem-solving process, and because nurses are trained in the nursing process (a problem-solving process), most perioperative advanced practice nurses already possess the skills required to formulate questions for integrative reviews. However, the skill, expertise, and research acumen required to carry out a secondary research literature review that will meet primary research scientific standards for rigor and replicability require education, training, and practice.

The integrative review

In 1982, Cooper [35] introduced scientific guidelines for conducting integrative research reviews. These guidelines were refined in a subsequent 1998 publication on research synthesis, where Cooper wrote that integrative research (research synthesis) focuses on "empirical studies and seeks to summarize past research, by drawing overall conclusions from many separate investigations that address related or identical hypotheses" [7]. In presenting guidelines for the scientific review, Cooper identified five stages for synthesizing research: (1) problem formulation; (2) data collection; (3) data evaluation; (4) analysis and interpretation, and (5) presentation.

In the problem formulation stage, decisions are made about what literature to review. Activities in this stage involve identifying the problem and operationalizing variables and concepts [35]. Cooper identifies threat to validity as a major concern for this stage and recommends that these threats be avoided by constructing the broadest possible conceptual definitions. The second stage of research synthesis, data collection or literature search, consists of determining which procedures should be used to find relevant literature and deciding which sources of potentially relevant literature to retrieve [7]. In establishing scientific guidelines for identifying potentially relevant sources, Cooper discusses issues related to rigor, validity, and replication. He recommends that, when conducting the secondary research review, the synthesists be explicit about the identification and selection of relevant literature by including information on the reference databases searched, the years covered by the search, the search terms, and the criteria used to determine what literature to retrieve for evaluation. In the data evaluation stage, evaluative standards are applied to the literature determined to meet the criteria for retrieval, to establish if the "evidence" contained in the retrieved document is valid or applicable to the problem focus. In this third stage of the synthesis process, Cooper recommends that potential issues with rigor, validity, and replication be addressed first of all by using a synthesis coding sheet that guides the retrieval of information from all documents "that might have the remotest possibility of

being considered relevant" [7]. At a minimum, the coding sheet should prompt the synthesists to record information relating to document identification and retrieval (authors, source of document, title, publication information, information leading to discovery of the document [search terms, and so forth]), and summary statements outlining key elements of the document's content (purpose, sample, setting, methodology, and so forth). Cooper also recommends that more than one "coder" examine each document, and that coders be trained in evaluation procedures to minimize unreliable retrieval of information from the documents. Intercoder agreement should be documented and reported, and "codes that lead to disagreement or low confidence should be discussed by multiple parties" involved in the review process [7]. In the fourth stage, analysis and interpretation, the focus of activity is synthesizing valid retrieved documents [7]. To ensure that the validity of interpretative conclusions can be evaluated by readers of the review, Cooper recommends that synthesists be as explicit as possible in determining and communicating interpretation rules [7]. In the fifth and final phase, presentation, Cooper identifies one potential source of invalidation of review conclusions to be the failure to communicate the procedures used to conduct the review. Therefore, to increase replicability, the synthesists should clearly delineate all steps and procedures used to identify, organize, and synthesize the literature. Although Cooper did not identify a standard set of research process tools for use in each of the research synthesis stages, he consistently emphasized the value of standardization and rigor in identifying (problem formulation, data collection), organizing (data evaluation), and synthesizing (analyzing and interpretation) literature for the research review.

Ganong built on the early work of Cooper and expanded the discussion related to methods and procedures for adding rigor and replicability to the integrative interview. Ganong [14] conducted an analysis of integrative reviews published in leading nursing journals between 1978 and 1983, to determine if the publications met a set of proposed criteria for a research review. Seventeen articles were examined on 12 dimensions: "purpose statements, sampling method, criteria for inclusion of studies, characteristics of primary research identified, citations of previous reviews, critique of previous reviews, presentation of primary research findings, method of analyzing results, discussion of methodological problems, search for systematic influences, interpretation of results, and use of tables" [14]. Ganong acknowledged that, even though a limited number of studies were analyzed, the number of published secondary research reviews included in the sample was sufficient to determine that the studies did not meet the standards for rigor and replicability common to primary research. Specifically, Ganong found that purpose statements were poorly articulated; sampling procedures were not clearly explained; pertinent characteristics of the literature review were not discussed; standards for analysis and interpretation were not made clear; and the reporting of results was vague. Ganong concluded that, even though methods for conducting integrative reviews vary, readers of these secondary research reviews should be able to identify principles of rigor associated with several standard steps. These standard steps are depicted in Table 1 and are matched with the five stages for synthesis identified by Cooper [7] and presented earlier in this article.

Stetler and colleagues [16] also addressed the issue of rigor and reliability in the integrative research review. While preparing to conduct an integrative review to support the development of a practice guideline, this group of nurses discovered that available frameworks for conducting the integrative review did not provide sufficient detail and direction. In response to this identified gap, Stetler and colleagues outlined an integrative review process and identified several recommendations for increasing the rigor and replicability of integrative reviews. These recommendations are presented in Table 1, along with similar recommendations made by Whittemore and Knafl [11]. In an article written to distinguish the integrative review from other research review methods, Whittemore and Knafl proposed methodologic strategies to enhance the rigor of the integrative review process.

The five-stage integrative literature review depicted in Table 1 can be used to evaluate the state of the science related to a specific research, policy, or practice topic; identify gaps in current research; identify a theoretic or conceptual framework; and identify research methods that demonstrate scientific rigor [36]. Great' progress has been made in increasing the rigor and replicability required to validate the yield of evidence from this type of research review. However, inconsistencies and variations in application of the published recommendations for increasing rigor and replicability continue to exist in the published literature, raising questions about the trustworthiness of evidence determined using the integrative research review. The IOS strategy presented in this article was developed to promote research- and evidence-based practice and to address the concerns related to rigor and replication of the integrative review that have been identified in the nursing literature. Through standardization of a specific set of process tools used to identify (problem formulation, data collection and literature search), organize (data evaluation), and synthesize (data analysis and interpretation) literature, the yield of evidence determined through use of the integrative review can be evaluated to determine the strength of rigor and replicability associated with the review process.

The identifying, organizing, and synthesizing strategy

Table 2 provides an overview of the IOS strategy and process steps in relation to the five-stage research synthesis process, the research process, and the synthesis of major recommendations for increasing rigor and replicability associated with the integrative review. The IOS strategy is a compilation of the steps of the research synthesis and research processes; and the set of standardized IOS process tools are conceived based on the major recommendations for rigor and replicability presented in Table 1.

A protocol is a written plan of study. Protocols are used to support the research and integrative review processes and to provide a mechanism to ensure that the steps of these processes are performed in a well-organized, logical, focused, and proficient manner [3–6,8,18]. The major research process steps or components of the research protocol are outlined in Table 2. These components are thoroughly explained in many research textbooks, several of which are included as references in this article. Readers are referred to a textbook on nursing research for a detailed explanation of each step. The major components for an integrative review protocol are also depicted in Table 2. For a detailed explanation of these steps, refer to references by Cooper, Ganong, Stetler and colleagues, or Whittemore and Knafl [11,14,16,19,35]. Detailed explanations of each IOS protocol step and the corresponding process tools are presented here.

Table 1
Stages of research synthesis and recommendations from the nursing literature for increasing rigor and replicability of the integrative research review

Cooper's stages of research synthesis [7]	Ganong recommendations [14]	Stetler et al recommendations [16]	Whittemore and Knafl recommendations [11]
Problem formulation	Formulate the purpose and develop research questions to be answered by the review.	Form a review team of interested nurses (stakeholders and individuals knowledgeable in research use). Determine the purpose of the review.	Formulate a well-specified research purpose to facilitate accurate operationalization of variables and extraction of data.
Data collection or literature search	Establish criteria for inclusion of studies in the review. Conduct the literature search, making sampling decisions if the number of studies identified is too large.	Identify key search terms and sources for the search. Develop a set of criteria to guide extraction of data. Pilot and refine criteria. Elect credible studies for inclusion in the review.	Clearly document the search process, including search terms, databases for the search, and inclusion and exclusion criteria.
Data evaluation	Develop a questionnaire to be used in gathering data from the studies.	Critique and record the facts or evidence from each study. Use evidence summary tables to record key details and provide quick review of data. Critique and record review of studies individually; each study should have at least two readers. Use consensus of two readers, and a third reader if necessary, to facilitate final recording of data.	Code documents reviewed on methodologic or theoretic rigor and relevance.
Analysis and interpretation	Identify rules of inference for data analysis and interpretation. Analyze data systematically. Discuss and interpret data.	Involve the review team in analysis, interpretation, and decision making. Provide each team member with a synopsis of all studies reviewed in preparation for synthesis discussions. Synthesize findings and evaluate applicability using a predetermined method. Develop recommendations.	Identify a systematic method for analyzing the data before initiating the review, to include data reduction, data display, data comparison, and drawing conclusions and verification.
Presentation of results	Report the review clearly and completely.		Report conclusions in table or diagrammatic format. Report all methodologic limitations.

Data from Refs [7,11,14,16].

Table 2
Stages of research synthesis, research process steps, synthesis of recommendations for rigor and replication, and identifying, organizing, and synthesizing strategy and tools

Stage in the research synthesis process	Corresponding research process steps	Synthesis for rigor and replication	IOS strategy steps and tools
Problem formulation	Problem identification Statement of purpose Formulation of aims	Use of review team of clinical and research experts Clearly constructed statement of purpose Clear identification of key concepts	Identifying: Formulation of the problem Statement of purpose Construction of clear research question Identification of key concepts and major search terms Process tools: Reviewers: a team of clinical/research process experts
Data collection or literature search	Research design Sample and sampling techniques Methods of measurement	Rigorous, replicable, written plan for data collection and data analysis Clear identification of inclusion/exclusion criteria Interreviewer reliability in conducting search	Identifying: Selection of studies for inclusion in the sample Definition of inclusion and exclusion criteria Conduction of the systematic search using pairs and group consensus Process tools: Reviewers Search algorithm
Data evaluation	Data collection	Use of pilot-tested data extraction tool to record evidence from each study Use of summary tables to record key details from each study Use of consensus of at least two readers in making evaluative decisions	Organizing: Uniform extraction of findings from studies included in the sample of documents Summary of studies included in the sample of literature documents Process tools: Reviewers Document review template Sample summary table

Analysis and interpretation	Data analysis	Use of a systematic method for analyzing the data Use of summary tables to reduce, display, and compare data	Synthesizing: Synthesis of extracted data Clear presentation of synthesis of data from each study Process tools: Reviewers Analysis and interpretation summary table Annotated bibliography
Presentation of results	Dissemination of findings	Clearly presented recommendations Discussion of methodologic limitations	Synthesizing: Presentation of results Discussion of methodologic limitations Recommendations for practice, policy, or research Suggestions for additional reviews

Data from Refs. [3–8,11,14,16,18].

Identifying, organizing, and synthesizing strategy: identifying

Formulating the problem

In the research and integrative review processes, the problem is the area of concern or the perplexing situation where a gap exists in the knowledge base needed for practice [3,5,8,18,37]. The purpose is a declarative statement that identifies the goal of the study or integrative review, whereas the research question is an interrogative statement that indicates what specifically will be sought out in the problem or area of concern. The purpose statement includes the variables of interest, population of interest, and an action verb, whereas the research question is written in the present tense and includes the variables and population of interest. Thus, most purpose statements can be reworded as research questions [3,5].

Process tool

The recommended process tool for the first step and each subsequent step of the IOS strategy is a team of clinical and research experts who serve as the reviewers who begin the integrative review process by formulating a problem that addresses "what," "who," and "why"; a statement of purpose that addresses "how"; and the research question that indicates "what specifically." An example of how the purpose and research question might be worded is presented in Box 1, along with a description of the composition of the team of reviewers. The research question selected for use in Box 1 has been purposely narrowed to facilitate its use as an example for application of all of the IOS process tools.

Selection of studies for inclusion in the sample

Inclusion criteria are sampling requirements that must be present for the document to be included in the sample of literature, and exclusion criteria are sampling requirements that eliminate a document from being in the literature sample. In the IOS strategy, the construction of inclusion and exclusion criteria begins with the definition of major terms in the research question. Once terms are clearly defined, decisions can be made about key words that will be used to guide the literature search. Once these decisions have been made by the team of reviewers, other decisions can be made that include type of documents to retrieve (research only, primary integrative reviews, integrative reviews of integrative reviews); year parameters for the search; types and number of

Box 1. Example of reviewer team, purpose statement, and research question

Reviewers
Four perioperative clinical nurse specialist students with a combined 23 years of experience in the perioperative clinical setting; one perioperative nurse specialist with 10 years in the perioperative clinical setting; one doctorally prepared nurse with 8 years of experience with the research process.

Statement of purpose
To determine if integrative research reviews published in the perioperative nursing literature between 1998 and 2007 meet a proposed set of standards for rigor and replication.

Research question
Do integrative research reviews published in the perioperative nursing literature between 1998 and 2007 meet a proposed set of standards for rigor and replication?

bibliographic databases to be used in conducting the search; and language restrictions for the literature documents, (ie, English language only).

Process tools

In addition to the team of reviewers, the process tools for this phase of the IOS strategy include a literature search algorithm. Fig. 1 is a depiction of what the search algorithm might look like after it has been constructed, refined, and used by the team of reviewers. Fig. 1 includes the purpose statement identified for use as an example from Box 1, inclusion and exclusion criteria for the search, key search terms, and actual search results. The following IOS steps outline the strategies for selecting studies for inclusion in the sample.

1. Creation of a search algorithm using the inclusion and exclusion criteria decided on by the team of reviewers.
2. Training of the team of reviewers to ensure consistent use of the algorithm when it is tested and implemented.
3. Testing of the algorithm to ensure consistent use of the tool by the reviewers and to

identify additional and optimal key search words. Process for testing the algorithm is as follows: One bibliographic database and one target search year is selected and all reviewer team members independently conduct a search using the criteria and parameters outlined in the algorithm. Each team member makes observations in a "search journal" related to the usefulness of the algorithm and identification of additional search terms. Abstracts and or articles are not retrieved during this testing of the algorithm.

4. Refinement of the algorithm consists of comparing team member observations during the test of the algorithm, and expanding key word search terms and phrases as appropriate.
5. Conducting the search using the algorithm. To increase credibility, dependability, and confirmability of the search [6,38], at least two members of the team are assigned to conduct a search on each database using the key words and search strategy outlined in the search algorithm. Studies identified during the search are evaluated for relevance to the research question based on the information included in the title, abstract, and key descriptor terms. Abstracts of relevant published studies are obtained, annotated with key words used to locate the abstract, and organized by year published. Each pair of team members should confirm the results of its search by comparing abstracts obtained with the algorithm search criteria.
6. Determining which abstracts meet the criteria for inclusion in the sample. After confirmation of the search among each pair of the research team, each set of abstracts is brought back to the review team to eliminate duplicate abstracts and to validate that each retained abstract meets the inclusion criteria for the literature sample. Once the team of reviewers has verified the results of the search, the published study corresponding to each abstract is obtained.

Identifying, organizing, and synthesizing strategy: organizing

Uniform extraction of findings from studies included in the sample

To minimize variance and increase the precision of data extraction, a data collection, or

Search Algorithm Example

Research question: Do integrative literature reviews published in the perioperative nursing literature meet a proposed set of standards for rigor and replication?

Inclusion Criteria: All primary and secondary integrative review articles or summaries related to perioperative nursing practice with abstracts, and published in the English language; retrieved using the keywords indicated below; human research only

Exclusion Criteria: Articles or theoretical papers on how to conduct an integrative review; systematic reviews of the literature

Name of Bibliographic Search Source: Pub Med (National Library of Medicine)

Year Searched: 1998-2007 **Date of Search**: 10/01/07 **Person Conducting Search:** _____

Exploration Using Preliminary Search Terms: Conduct a preliminary search using the search terms listed below to determine the number of hits returned for each term, assess the scope and appropriateness of search terms, and to identify other potential literature search terms. Enter search terms as they appear below. Record the number of hits on this form and annotate observations relating to duplicate articles, scope of articles returned for each set of terms, and proposed additional terms in your literature search journal.

Number of Hits on Search Terms	Search Terms
6	Perioperative nursing AND Integrative review
6	Perioperative nursing AND Integrative research
4	Perioperative nursing AND "Integrative review" of literature
2	Perioperative nursing AND "Integrated review" of literature
3	Perioperative nursing AND Literature synthesis
5	Perioperative nursing AND Research synthesis

Fig. 1. Search algorithm example. [1]A primary integrative literature review is a summary and analysis of previous empiric or theoretic literature to provide a broader understanding of a phenomenon of interest [3,7,11,17]. Other terms used to describe the integrative review include literature or literature synthesis. A secondary integrative review is an integrative review of a set of published integrative reviews. Articles or theoretic papers on how to conduct a literature review are excluded. Systematic reviews of the literature are excluded. Abstracts containing the phrase "literature review" but not containing the terms "integrated," integrative, research synthesis, or literature synthesis are excluded. [2]"Perioperative Nursing Related" includes perioperative, operating room, perianesthesia, and postanesthesia.

Search and Abstract Retrieval: Conduct the search using the key words below and the search algorithm. Annotate and save those abstracts determined to meet inclusion criteria documented on the form and in the search algorithm below. Keep careful journal notes about use of and justification for additional search terms. Save abstracts to the clipboard or a literature reference management program for review.

Number of Hits	Number of Abstracts Saved	Duplicate Save	Search Terms
6	1	0	Perioperative nursing AND Integrative review
6	1	1	Perioperative nursing AND Integrative research
4	0	0	Perioperative nursing AND "Integrative review" of literature
2	1	1	Perioperative nursing AND "Integrated review" of literature
3	1	1	Perioperative nursing AND Literature synthesis
5	1	1	Perioperative nursing AND Research synthesis

- Use the following algorithm to determine which abstracts to save and annotate. If abstracts appear under more than one set of search terms save the abstract once but annotate with all applicable search terms and record as a duplicate save and under number of abstracts saved.

  - Begin Review
    - Integrative Review of the Literature[1]
      - Yes—Continue Review
      - No—Discard
    - Perioperative Nursing Related[2]?
      - No—Discard
      - Yes—Save abstract and annotate with the Key Words used for search

---

[1]A primary integrative literature review is a summary and analysis of previous empirical and/or theoretical literature to provide a broader understanding of a phenomenon of interest [3,7,11,17]. Other terms used to describe the integrative review include literature or literature synthesis. A secondary integrative review is an integrative review of a set of published integrative reviews. Articles or theoretical papers on how to conduct a literature review are excluded. Systematic reviews of the literature are excluded. Abstracts containing the phrase "literature review" but not containing the terms "integrated", integrative, research synthesis, or literature synthesis are excluded.
[2] "Perioperative Nursing Related" includes perioperative, OR, perianesthesia and postanesthesia.

Fig. 1 (*continued*)

coding, sheet is developed to guide extraction of data. Because each extraction tool is specific to each question or problem focus, the review template is developed by the review team with the assistance of experts in the research process.

Various quantitative and qualitative methods have been adapted for use in the extraction of data during secondary research reviews. However, because the integrative review includes empiric and theoretic literature, manifest content analysis

Sample Document Review Template for Review of Integrative Literature Reviews Published in the Perioperative Nursing Literature

Document Review Template ID Number _____

Reviewer _____

Section 1: Search Information:

A. Search Date (Month and Year): _____

B. Key Words Used (Write in all that apply):

C. Timeframe of Search (Years Covered): _____ .

D. Where was the document located at MEDLINE, CINAHL, or BOTH? Circle the correct CHOICE or

    write in not applicable._____

Section 2: Document Information:

A. Title of the document_____..._____

B. Author (s):_____..._____

C. WRITTEN Purpose of the Document:

D. Research Question addressed in the review:

E. What are the WRITTEN major variables of interest identified in the document?

Section 3: Document Evaluation

A. Is the source of the integrative research review?

Peer reviewed scientific journal	_____ Yes	_____ No	_____ Unknown
Annual review of research publication	_____ Yes	_____ No	_____ Unknown
Unpublished dissertation or thesis	_____ Yes	_____ No	_____ Unknown

B. Is the practice problem clearly defined?   _____ Yes   _____ No   _____ Unknown

        Formulation of the problem
- Statement of purpose
- Construction of clear research question
- Identification of key concepts and major search terms

C. Were a team of Reviewers utilized to conduct the research review of the literature?

        _____ Yes   _____ No   _____ Unknown

    If yes, what is the composition of the team?_____..._____

D. Was a written protocol developed to guide the research review process?

        _____ Yes   _____ No   _____ Unknown

Fig. 2. Sample document review template for review of integrative literature reviews published in the perioperative nursing literature.

E. Was a sufficient number of studies included in the research review?

        Yes   No   Unknown

- o Number of relevant studies found/number cited:_____
- o Number of studies included in the summary/synthesis tables:_____

F. Are the procedures used to derive the sample clearly described and systematic?

        Yes   No   Unknown

- o Selection of studies for inclusion in the sample
- o Definition of inclusion and exclusion criteria
- o Conduction of the systematic search

G. Are the data extraction/coding procedures clearly described and uniformed across all studies reviewed?

        Yes   No   Unknown

H. Are the criteria used to analyze/synthesize data clearly defined and consistent across all studies?

        Yes   No   Unknown

I. Are findings from the analysis presented in a clear and organized manner?

        Yes   No   Unknown

- o Use of summary tables
- o Use of annotated bibliographies
- o Sufficient detail for evaluation by the reader

J. Are methodological limitations for the research review clearly addressed?

        Yes   No   Unknown

K. What type of recommendations are concluded in the review?

      Practice   Research   Other   None

What are the recommendations_____..._____

K. What is the strength of the recommendations from this research review?

      High   Low   Unknown

- o Formed around the major concepts generating the review
- o Based on evidence derived from the integrative review
- o Clinical and statistical significance are addressed
- o Studies included in the review are recent

K. Does this integrative review meet the standards for rigor and replicability required for secondary research reviews?

        Yes   No   Unknown

Justification for the response_____..._____

Fig. 2 (*continued*)

Table 3
Abbreviated sample summary example: integrative research reviews published in the perioperative nursing literature between 1998 and 2007

Authors and bibliographic information	Title	Bibliographic database used	Key search words for document retrieval	Purpose	Sample
Armstrong & Bortz 2001 [40]	An integrative review of pressure relief in surgical patients	PubMed	Perioperative nursing and integrative review; perioperative nursing and integrative research	To determine if pressure-relieving support surfaces significantly reduce intraoperative tissue pressure and result in a lower incidence of postoperative pressure ulcers	22 studies meeting inclusion criteria
Fallis 2002 [41]	Monitoring bladder temperature in the operating room	PubMed	Perioperative nursing and integrated review of literature; perioperative nursing and literature synthesis; perioperative nursing and research synthesis	To provide a systematic, integrated review and synthesis of research related to bladder temperature monitoring in the operating room	12 studies meeting search criteria
Fetzer & Hand 2001 [42]	A profile of perianesthesia nursing patient outcome research, 1994–1999	PubMed	Perioperative nursing and integrative research	To profile the current body of perianesthesia nursing research and extend findings of pervious integrative review completed for 1982 to 1993	31 studies appearing in 18 specific journals related to perianesthesia

Table 4
Abbreviated analyses and interpretation summary table for integrative research reviews published in the perioperative nursing literature

Authors	Purpose	Major concepts used in literature search	Composition of review team	Sample	Sampling methodology	Data extraction tools
Armstrong & Bortz (2001) [40]	To determine if pressure-relieving support surfaces significantly reduce intraoperative tissue pressure and result in a lower incidence of postoperative pressure ulcers	Skin breakdown, surgery, skin integrity, research, perioperative, Braden Scale, Hemphill's Guidelines for Assessment of Pressure Sore Potential, Modified Knoll Assessment Tool, operating room, risk factors, mattresses and pads, support surfaces, intraoperative complications, pressure sores, pressure ulcers	Not described	22 studies meeting inclusion criteria	Search and inclusion criteria are clearly identified; date parameters for search are identified; researchers purposively selected studies meeting the search criteria; electronic and manual searches of the literature were conducted	Not described
Fallis (2002) [41]	To provide a systematic, integrated review and synthesis of research related to bladder temperature monitoring in the operating room	Body temperature, bladder, esophageal, nasopharyngeal, pulmonary artery, operating room, and surgery	Not described	12 studies meeting search criteria	Search and inclusion criteria are clearly identified; date parameters for search are not identified; sampling methodology is not described	Not described
Fetzer & Hand (2001) [42]	To profile the current body of perianesthesia nursing research and extend findings of previous integrative review completed for 1982 to 1993	Perianesthesia, ambulatory surgery, postanesthesia, day surgery	Two nurse researchers	31 studies appearing in 18 specific journals between 1982 to 1993 and related to perianesthesia	Search and inclusion criteria are clearly identified; date parameters for search are identified; studies were purposively selected by two nurse researchers independently; electronic and manual searches of the literature were conducted; consensus was reached for studies included in the sample	Modified version of the Ambulatory Post Anesthesia Research Literature Instrument

has been adopted as the primary analysis method in the IOS strategy and as the framework for construction of the data extraction tool.

Content analysis is "a deductive process that involves looking for specific instances of narrative data to fit or illustrate a predetermined content area or theme" [5]. Although content analysis can be used to analyze interview transcripts associated with qualitative research studies, it is used more frequently to analyze more structured items such as documents, records, and policies [5,39]. Latent content analysis focuses on the meaning behind words, whereas manifest content analysis concentrates on the occurrence of specific key words, phrases, or characteristics. In the IOS strategy, manifest content analysis guides the construction of a precoded data collection tool used to guide the review of empiric and theoretic literature during the data evaluation phase of the integrative review. The data collection sheet is referred to as a document review template in the IOS strategy. Fig. 2 is an example of a document review template developed for use in the application example introduced in an earlier section of this article. The review template is tested and refined by the research team before being fully implemented. The procedural steps recommended for creating and refining the search algorithm are also used to test the review template.

Data extraction is performed by two independent reviewer team members. The pair of data extractors conducts a joint comparative review of both sets of completed document review templates. A reconciled, single set of the templates is presented to the entire team. If consensus cannot be reached by the two data extractors, a third reviewer is included.

Summary of studies included in the sample

A sample summary table is used to summarize and describe the major characteristics of the documents selected for inclusion in the sample. The purpose of this table is descriptive rather than analytic. The summary provides a quick reference for the review team of all the documents included in the sample. At a minimum, the headings of the table should include author or authors, title, bibliographic information, source of document, key words used to locate the document, purpose of the document, sample size, and comments. Additional headings are added as appropriate. Tables 3 and 4 provide an example of an abbreviated sample summary table and analyses tables

for the literature search conducted in the application example "to determine if integrative research reviews published in the perioperative nursing literature between 1998 and 2007 meet a proposed set of standards for rigor and replication."

Identifying, organizing, and synthesizing strategy: synthesizing

Clear and uniform presentation of data from each document and interpretation of results

In this phase of the IOS strategy, review team members use the sample summary table and completed document review templates to create an analysis and interpretation summary table. The analysis and interpretation summary table contains the content extracted from all the documents included in the review. In addition, a synthesis of the content of the analysis and interpretation table is placed in narrative text in the form of an annotated bibliography. An annotated bibliography is a descriptive and evaluative summary of a literature source [43]. The annotated bibliography is used in the IOS strategy to compare, contrast, and critique each literature source in terms providing evidence to answer the research question. In the IOS strategy, the annotated bibliography represents the review team's consensus and synthesis of content from the sample of documents in relation to relevance, accuracy, quality, rigor, and replicability. Additionally, in the final phase of the IOS strategy, presentation of the results is concentrated on discussion of methodologic limitations and recommendations for practice, policy, or research.

Summary

The vision for perioperative nursing in the 21st century is validation of professional practice, maintenance of identity and credibility as a discipline, substantiation of accountability for the quality of care delivered, and integration of research as a means of providing evidence for practice (see Refs. [20,21,28,44–46]). Actualization of this vision requires that perioperative nurses become active players in the journey, questioning every element of perioperative practice, gathering data, analyzing findings, implementing change to improve practice, evaluating outcomes associated with the change, and facilitating the change process required for widespread implementation of evidence-based practice [28].

"Practice cannot be justified on the basis of anecdotal experience or commercial interests; it must be evaluated by its influence on the outcome of surgical procedures and supported by scientific facts" [33]. By asking the question "why" and not settling for unresearched solutions, perioperative nurses can make a positive difference in the delivery of care for the surgical patient [34]. Ultimately, research generates knowledge and provides the scientific base to inform decisions and validate practices. Research to support evidence-based practice can be used to examine practices for efficiency, efficacy, and positive outcomes (patient specific or process focused) in an effort to discover the best available scientific evidence related to patient care delivery. Finding the evidence to support practice is key, and using the IOS strategy and process tools to guide the integrative research review provides perioperative nurses with the mechanism for successfully orchestrating an important part of the 21st century vision, evidence-based practice.

References

[1] Straus SE, Richardson WS, Glasziou P, et al. Evidence-based medicine: how to practice and teach EBM. 3rd edition. Edinburgh (Scotland): Churchill Livingstone; 2005.

[2] Fleschler R. Evidence-based practice. In: Fitzpatrick J, Wallace M, editors. Encyclopedia of nursing research. 2nd edition. New York: Springer; 2006. p. 183–5.

[3] Burns N, Grove SK. The practice of nursing research: conduct, critique, utilization. 5th edition. St Louis (MO): Elsevier Saunders; 2005.

[4] Gerrish K, Lacey A. The research process in nursing. 5th edition. Oxford (England): Blackwell; 2006.

[5] Norwood SL. Research strategies for advanced practice nurses. Upper Saddle River (NJ): Prentice Hall Health; 2000.

[6] Polit DF, Beck CT. Nursing research: principles and methods. Philadephia: Lipincott Williams & Wilkins; 2004.

[7] Cooper HM. Synthesizing research: a guide for literature reviews. 3rd edition. Thousand Oaks (CA): Sage; 1998.

[8] Higgins JPT, Green S. Cochrane handbook for systematic reviews of interventions 4.2.6. [updated September 2006]. In:Higgins JPT, Green S, editors. The Cochrane library, vol 4. Chichester (UK): John Wiley & Sons, Ltd.; 2006.

[9] Stevens KR. Systematic reviews: the heart of evidence based practice. AACN Clin Issues 2001; 12(4):529–38.

[10] Weaver K, Olsen JK. Integrative literature reviews and meta-analyses: understanding paradigm used for nursing research. J Adv Nurs 2006;53(4):459–69.

[11] Whittemore R, Knafl K. The integrative review: updated methodology. J Adv Nurs 2005;52(5): 546–53.

[12] Jones ML. Application of systematic review methods to qualitative research: practical issues. J Adv Nurs 2004;48(3):271–8.

[13] Beyea SC, Nicoll LH. Writing an integrative review. AORN J 1998;67(4):877–80.

[14] Ganong LH. Integrative reviews of nursing research. Res Nurs Health 1987;10:1–11.

[15] Goldsmith MR, Bankhead CR, Austoker J. Synthesizing quantitative and qualitative research in evidence-based patient information. J Epidemiol Community Health 2007;61:262–70.

[16] Stetler CB, Morsi D, Rucki S, et al. Utilization focused integrative reviews in nursing service. Appl Nurs Res 1998;11(4):195–205.

[17] Whittemore R. Combining evidence in nursing research: methods and implications. Nurs Res 2005; 54(1):56–62.

[18] Hulley SB, Newman TB, Cummings SR. Getting started: the anatomy and physiology of clinical research. In: Hulley SB, Cummings SR, Browner WS, et al, editors. Designing clinical research. 2nd edition. Philadelphia: Lippincott Williams and Wilkins; 2001. p. 3–15.

[19] Cooper H. A taxonomy of literature reviews. Psychol Bull 2003;129(1):3–9.

[20] Bailes B. Evidence-based practice guidelines–one way to enhance clinical practice. AORN J 2002; 75(6):1166–7.

[21] Beyea S. Why should perioperative RNs care about evidence-based practice? AORN J 2000;72(1): 109–11.

[22] Beyea S. Clinical practice guidelines–an organizational effort. AORN J 2000;71(4):852, 855–8.

[23] Lipp A. The systematic review as an evidence-based tool for the operating room. AORN J 2005;81(6): 1279–80.

[24] Beyea S. Evidence-based practice in perioperative nursing. Am J Infect Control 2004;32:247–80.

[25] Ervin N. Evidence-based nursing practice: are we there yet? J N Y State Nurses Assoc 2002;33(2):11–6.

[26] Magarey JM. Elements of a systematic review. Int J Nurs Pract 2001;7:376–82.

[27] Hakesley-Brown R. No cutting corners in cutting edge care. Journal of Advanced Perioperative Care 2002;1(1):3 [Chairman's Message].

[28] O'Reilly D. An analysis of perioperative care. Br J Perioper Nurs 2001;11(9):402–11.

[29] Csokasy J. Building perioperative nursing research teams–part I. AORN J 1997;65(2):396–401.

[30] Distler JW. Critical thinking and clinical competence: results of the implementation of student centered teaching strategies in an advanced practice nurse curriculum. Nurse Educ Pract 2007;7(1): 53–9.

[31] Profetto-McGrath J, Smith KB, Hugo K, et al. Clinical nurse specialists' use of evidence in

practice: a pilot study. Worldviews on Evidence Based Nursing 2007;4(2):86–96.

[32] Association of periOperative Registered Nurses. Introduction to 2007 edition. In: Standards, recommended practices, and guidelines. Denver (CO): AORN; 2007. p. v-vi.

[33] Belkin N. Masks, barriers, laundering, and gloving: where is the evidence? AORN J 2006;84(4):655–7 660–4.

[34] Girard N. Never underestimate the importance of asking "why?" AORN J 2005;82(6):961–2.

[35] Cooper HM. Scientific guidelines for conducting integrative research reviews. Rev Educ Res 1982;52: 291–302.

[36] Russell CL. An overview of the integrative research review. Prog Transplant 2005;15(1):8–13.

[37] Lacey A. The research process. In: Gerrish K, Lacey A, editors. The research process in nursing. 5th edition. Oxford: Blackwell; 2006. p. 16–30.

[38] Hearst N, Grady D, Barron HV, et al. Research using existing data: secondary data analysis, ancillary studies, and systematic reviews. In: Hulley SB, Cummings SR, Browner WS, editors. Designing clinical research. 2nd edition. Philadelphia: Lippincott Williams and Wilkins; 2001. p. 195–212.

[39] Bowling A. Research methods in health: investigating health and health services. 2nd edition. Maidenhead (UK): Open University Press; 2002.

[40] Armstrong D, Bortz P. An integrative review of pressure relief in surgical patients. AORN J 2001; 73(3):645, 647–8.

[41] Fallis WM. Monitoring bladder temperatures in the OR. AORN J 2002;76(3):467–76; 481–4,486, 488–9.

[42] Fetzer SJ, Hand MC. A profile of perianesthesia patient outcome research, 1994–1999. J PeriAnesth Nurs 2001;16(5):315–24.

[43] Cornell University Library. How to prepare an annotated bibliography. Available at: http://www.library.cornell.edu/olinuris/ref/research/skill28.htm. Accessed 20 August, 2007.

[44] Dean A, Fawcett T. Nurses' use of evidence in preoperative fasting. Nurs Stand 2002;17(12):33–7.

[45] Michael R. Facilitating nursing research. Australian College of Operating Room Nursing (ACORN) Journal 2006;19(1):18–22.

[46] Osborne S, Gardner G. Imperatives and strategies for developing an evidence-based practice in perioperative nursing. Australian College of Operating Room Nurses Journal (ACORN) 2004;17(1): 18–24.

ELSEVIER
SAUNDERS

Perioperative Nursing Clinics 3 (2008) 19–26

PERIOPERATIVE
NURSING
CLINICS

Florence Nightingale, Dr. Ernest Codman, American College of Surgeons Hospital Standardization Committee, and The Joint Commission: Four Pillars in the Foundation of Patient Safety

Charlotte M. Shell, MSN, RN[a],*,
Karen D. Dunlap, MSN, RN, CNOR[b]

[a]Brooke Army Medical Center, 3851 Roger Brooke Drive, Fort Sam Houston, TX 78234-6200, USA
[b]Walter Reed Army Medical Center, 6900 Georgia Avenue NW, Washington, DC 20307, USA

For us who Nurse, our Nursing is a thing, unless in it we are making progress every year, every month, every week, take my word for it, we are going back.

> —Florence Nightingale [1]

Patient safety, performance improvement, and quality care are familiar terms in today's health care industry. The Hippocratic principle of "First, do no harm" is ingrained in all the disciplines. Yet every year, patients needlessly fall prey to substandard care and medical errors that have the capacity to cause catastrophic injury and even death.

The relationship among substandard care, medical errors, and medical care is not simply a dilemma associated with the advanced technologies of the twentieth century. Back in 1854, during the Crimean War, Florence Nightingale assumed the position of "superintendent of the female nursing establishment of the English general hospitals" in Turkey. While in this role, she collected data on mortality rates of soldiers. She divided her data into three categories: (1) deaths caused by preventable contagious diseases, (2) deaths due to the patient's wounds, and (3) deaths from all other causes. Nightingale soon realized soldiers were dying as patients in field hospitals from avoidable complications and

pathology at a faster rate than those dying on the battlefield. As a result of her findings, she implemented actions to improve standards of care, and the death rate fell dramatically.

Fifty-six years later, in 1910, the idea of assessing patient outcomes was revisited by Ernest Codman, MD. This novel thought process, called the "end result system of standardization," suggested that hospitals track patient care outcomes for all patients admitted [2,3]. Successful outcomes would indicate treatments should be repeated for similar cases, whereas failures would reveal a need for a different treatment regimen. Although several of his colleagues agreed with his end result idea, the medical community at large did not support the capturing of data they felt could be disheartening to the public and negatively impact hospitals and providers. A determined Codman continued to support his end result idea and in 1911 opened his own 20-bed hospital, in which he meticulously collected outcomes data on all his patients. Committed to increasing patient safety, Codman published his findings in his hospital's report, and encouraged the professional community to do the same. In hopes that others would emulate his actions, he gave prominent hospitals a copy of the report, which clearly identified his successes and errors. To the surprise of many, Codman even gave his report to prospective patients without expressing fear of the consequences of his actions [4,5].

As crusaders for quality care, Nightingale (1820–1910) and Codman (1869–1940) may well

---

* Corresponding author.

E-mail address: charlotte.shell@us.army.mil
(C.M. Shell).

1556-7931/08/$ - see front matter. Published by Elsevier Inc.
doi:10.1016/j.cpen.2007.11.004

deserve the credit for the birth of evidence-based medicine. One can only imagine the synergy they would have achieved in improving patient outcomes had they been afforded the opportunity to combine their efforts.

Institute of Medicine report (1999)

The 1999 Institute of Medicine report, "To Err Is Human," proved to be a pivotal impetus for our nation and motivated health care leaders to take action toward promoting patient safety and improving medical outcomes. The unimaginable volumes of medical errors identified within the report were supported by staggering statistics. Chapter two of the report states, "deaths in hospitals due to preventable adverse events exceed the number attributable to the 8th leading cause of death. Deaths due to preventable adverse events exceed the deaths attributable to motor vehicle accidents, breast cancer or AIDS....Although the risk of dying as a result of a medical error far surpassed the risk of dying in an airplane accident, a good deal more public attention has been focused on improving safety in the airline industry than in the health care industry. The likelihood of dying per domestic jet flight is estimated to be one in eight million. Statistically, an average passenger would have to fly around the clock for more than 438 years before being involved in a fatal crash" [6].

American College of Surgeons Hospital Standardization Committee and The Joint Commission

In 1912, at the New York Clinical Congress of Surgeons, the American College of Surgeons (ACS) announced the first ever Hospital Standardization Committee. Codman's "end result system" was one of its main objectives. In 1917, over a 3-day conference, ACS fellows, hospital superintendents, and committee members were challenged with discussing and identifying aspects to include in the minimum standard. In 1918, the Hospital Standardization Committee launched the first field testing of its one-page minimum standard (Fig. 1). Participants were shocked to learn that only 89 of the 692 100+ bed hospitals surveyed met all of the minimum standards. The results were absolutely dismal. Fearing adverse media coverage, the list of compliant hospitals was never distributed at the congress. Instead, the night before the conference, all records were burned in the furnace of the Waldorf-Astoria

Hotel; the public would never be given the opportunity to learn the truth [4,7].

By 1921, 76% of the surveyed hospitals scored compliant, and it was in this year that a formal list of compliant hospitals was published. By 1926, the minimum standard grew into the first *Manual of Hospital Standardization*, 18 pages in length. Smaller hospitals were being surveyed, along with the larger ones, to raise the number of surveys from 692 to more than 13,000. Over the next 20 years, the manual continued to grow, to 118 pages in length, with added expectations aimed at improving the standards of care [4].

In 1946, Congress acknowledged the value of the ACS surveys through the passing of the Hill-Burton Act. The act provided federal funding for hospital construction, but with the specification that the hospitals have ACS certification. As the credibility of the Hospital Standardization Program grew, the demands of sole financial burden for sustainment on the ACS continued to increase. In the search for a new sponsor, the ACS collaborated with the American Hospital Association, the American Medical Association, and the American College of Physicians to provide that support. After months of power and control struggles, the draft for a joint commission to include the Canadian Medical Association was written. In November of 1951, an independent, not-for-profit organization was created: the Joint Commission on Accreditation of Hospitals (JCAH) [4].

Because of the increasing number of hospitals seeking accreditation and the resulting increase in expenditures, the JCAH began charging for surveys in 1964. The cost per hospital was a flat rate of 60 dollars, plus an additional 1 dollar per hospital bed up to 250 beds [4].

Survey and standards changes over the years

Each new decade brought with it numerous changes in the JCAH. The early 1970s saw the focus of the standards change from requiring minimum standards to requiring optimal, achievable levels of quality. The late 1970s saw the collaboration of the College of American Pathologists and the JCAH to evaluate hospital laboratories, and the American Dental Association became a corporate member.

The changes in the 1980s were no less impressive. The accreditation cycle was increased to every 3 years for hospitals, psychiatric facilities, substance abuse programs, community mental health programs, and long-term care organization. The

The Minimum Standard:

1. That physicians and surgeons privileged to practice in the hospital be organized as a definite group or staff. Such organization has nothing to do with the question as to whether the hospital is "open" or "closed", nor need it affect the various existing types of staff organization. The word "staff" is here defined as the group of doctors who practice in the hospital inclusive of all groups such as the "regular staff," "the visiting staff," and the "associated staff".

2. That membership upon the staff be restricted to physicians and surgeons who are (a) full graduates of medicine in good standing and legally licensed to practice in their respective states or provinces (b) competent in their respective fields, and (c) worthy in character and in matters of professional ethics; that in this latter connection the practice of the division of fees, under any guise whatever, be prohibited.

3. That the staff initiate and, with the approval of the governing board of the hospital, adopt rules, regulations, and policies governing the professional work of the hospital; that these regulations, and policies specifically provide:
   a. That staff meetings be held at least once each month. (In large hospitals the departments may choose to meet separately.)
   b. That the staff review and analyze regular intervals their clinical experience in the various departments of the hospital, such as medicine, surgery, obstetrics, and the other specialties; the clinical records of patients, free and pay, to be the basis for such review and analysis.

4. That accurate and complete records be written for all patients and filed in an accessible manner in the hospital – a complete case record being one which included identification data, complaint, personal and family history, history of the present illness, physical examination, special examinations, such as consultations, clinical laboratory, X-ray and other examinations, provisional or working diagnosis, medical or surgical treatment, gross and microscopic pathological findings, progress notes, final diagnosis, condition on discharge, follow-up and, in case of death, autopsy findings.

5. That diagnostic and therapeutic facilities under competent supervision be available for the study, diagnosis, and treatment of patients, these to include at least (a) a clinical laboratory providing chemical, bacteriological, serological, and pathological services; (b) an X-ray department providing radiographic and fluoroscopic services.

Fig. 1. American College of Surgeons Hospital Standardization Committee's one-page minimum standard.

scope of services expanded to include hospice care organizations, home health care, and managed care. To reflect the increase in scope of services beyond hospitals, the name of the JCAH changed to the Joint Commission on Accreditation of Healthcare Organization (JCAHO). Along with the name change came an evolution in survey method; the tailored survey approach started in 1983 was augmented 4 years later with the advent of the agenda for change [3].

Transformation in various areas continued throughout the 1990s. The main emphasis of the new survey process was placed on actual organization performance. With the development of the Indicator Measurement System, an indicator-based monitoring system was launched. During this same time period, Quality Healthcare Resources, Inc., a not-for-profit consulting subsidiary, was established. Many health care staff will remember this time not so much for the shift in focus to performance improvement, but rather for the policy prohibiting smoking in the hospital. After major revisions were made to reflect the new emphasis on actual organization performance, the new accreditation manuals were published. The revised standards, effective in 1995, revealed the transition to performance-based standards structured around functions central to patient care [3].

Looking back over the first 7 years of the twenty-first century, one can see that the survey processes continued to evolve exponentially. Now 50 years old, The Joint Commission would witness its most eventful decade to date. Ushered in during this time frame were the national patient safety goals and the universal protocol. A 30-member Nursing Advisory Council was created in 2003 to address the existing nursing shortage facing our nation. The most notable innovation occurred with the launching of the Shared Visions–New Pathways initiative in 2004. Although surveys were already random and unannounced, the new tracer methodology required health care organizations to reframe their accreditation process. Although some viewed it as painful, this new survey method has proven to be the most influential survey method designed to date, with surprisingly widespread acceptance among the multitudes of health care organizations.

The year 2005 saw the devastating effects of hurricanes Katrina, Wilma, and Rita, with the JCAHO immersed in the tragedy that affected so many of its accredited hospitals and health care organizations. Responding to their needs, the JCAHO published "Standing Together: An Emergency Planning Guide for America's Communities." Since the occurrence of these tragedies, emergency planning has taken on a new life of its own, not only across the country, but under the purview of the joint commission.

As the twenty-first century has progressed, so has the growth of the JCAHO's scope of services. Not only were foster care, assisted living, office-based surgery, critical access hospitals, disease-specific care, organ transplant, and chronic kidney disease management added to its list of programs accredited or certified after 2000 but staffing agencies and durable medical equipment companies were also certified. With this expansion, the organization changed its name to the Joint Commission. This change represented an extension of services beyond health care organizations, and with the ever-increasing involvement of the JCAHO in the political arena, a name change representing the true nature of the organization was needed.

Sentinel event policy and ORYX

The sentinel event policy was established and later revised to encourage health care organizations to self-report these events and to scrutinize their root causes. The Joint Commission defines a sentinel event as "an unexpected occurrence involving death or serious physical or psychological injury, or the risk thereof" [8]. The purpose of the policy is to improve patient care, treatment, and services by analyzing why the sentinel event occurred. A thorough analysis of the event, or the root cause analysis, drives the development of an action plan to improve systems or processes, thereby reducing the risk of event recurrence. Evaluation of the plan's effectiveness is necessary to ensure that lessons learned are shared and the potential for reoccurrence is decreased, or that similar events do not recur.

Although surveyors do not review sentinel events already reported to The Joint Commission, should an unreported event be discovered during the survey process, it will be reported to the organization CEO and The Joint Commission. The event will be reviewed and follow-up is required as per the sentinel event policy.

The Joint Commission may become aware of a sentinel event through various sources. The most common conduit is the self-reporting of an event by the involved health care organization. Other sources include hospital employees, patients, families, and the media. Self-reporting of a sentinel event enables The Joint Commission to add the information to its database, composed of events occurring across the nation. The information in this database can help other organizations which may have similar policies and procedures actually avoid negative outcomes by acting on the lessons learned by others. Sentinel events repeatedly reported to The Joint Commission, or those of a serious nature and with the potential to occur in other organizations, often become the focus of national patient safety goals.

In 1997, ORYX: the next evolution in accreditation was initiated. The resultant measurement requirements were intended to help organizations with their improvement processes. By 1999, the first ORYX data from accredited organizations was reviewed by the JCAHO. Five priority measurement areas were recommended by the state hospital association and were approved. In 2002, the first set of "core" performance measures was collected. The Joint Commission and the Centers for Medicare and Medicaid Services (CMS) aligned their required measures in an effort to reduce the cost of data collection and reporting by organizations. These measures, called hospital quality measures, feed into the priority focus process, which, in turn, helps direct survey activities. The data from these measures are reported on

The Joint Commission's Quality Check Web site, which allows public consumers to compare the quality of hospitals against each other and against national data [3,9].

Tracer methodology

With the shift toward examining organizational performance, in 2004 The Joint Commission introduced tracer methodology for its on-site surveys. In the restructuring process, surveyors eliminated time spent on reviewing performance improvement storyboards and organizational policy documents. This major change afforded surveyors the opportunity to spend more time observing actual patient care and the processes involved in that care. Tracer methodology is defined as "an evaluation method in which surveyors select a patient, resident or client and use that individual's record as a road map to move through an organization to assess and evaluate the organization's compliance with selected standards and the organization's systems of providing care and services" [10]. Classically complex patients receiving high-risk procedures make ideal tracers. For example, a surgical orthopedic patient who has cardiovascular disease, diabetes, and renal disease currently receiving dialysis will enable the surveyor to review consult processes with observations of various clinics, and by speaking to several providers and the health care staff. Operative permits, anesthesia records, intraoperative documents, progress notes, and transfer orders are scrutinized. Surveyors will gladly don a "bunny suit" or change into scrubs to tour the operating room and question the processes that occur behind closed doors. Compliance with universal protocol, use of flash sterilizers, and care of grafts will notably be on the top of the surveyor's mental list. At any point, medication management could be explored, with examination of anesthesia carts, visits to the pharmacy, and discussions with staff related to processes focused on patient teaching. The tracer will continue in the dialysis unit where infection control methods, emergency responses, and equipment maintenance are reviewed with staff. Of course, this same patient tracer could lead the surveyor to the laboratory or medical maintenance. During the tracer, compliance with national patient safety goals are assessed and observed, which affords the opportunity to evaluate medication reconciliation, patient hand-offs, critical laboratory values, and hand hygiene. At every corner, occasions exist to evaluate observable safety measures. Approximately 60% of the surveyor's time is spent conducting tracers during his/her visit.

Tracer methodology has been a phenomenal success, as evidenced by surveyed organizations developing their own tracer teams. By conducting routine tracers, organizations are able to monitor their own standard of care and compliance with standards, quickly identify risk points, and address areas requiring system review and improvements.

Standards development

Most health care providers have, at one time or another, expressed skepticism or negative opinions about The Joint Commission's development of standards. The perception of arbitrary development, non–evidence-based decisions, and randomly selected, pulled-out-of-the-air standards are complaints heard from various health care providers. In actuality, nothing could be further from the truth. The complex process of standard development involves many sources and layers. It lies at the core of what The Joint Commission offers the world of patient safety and is one of its central tasks. Standard development is an ongoing, dynamic process that incorporates scientific literature and the experiences and perspectives of health care professionals, field experts, and professional organizations.

The development of a standard follows a specific process. The first step taken by the Joint Commission is to determine that a relevant need exists. Concerns are identified through various sources. Literature (such as the Institute of Medicine report), surveyor experiences, identified needs by experts and interest groups, changes in the environment (such as bioterrorism and natural disasters), legislation, and media are all sources of potential needs. Initial research is then performed by reviewing the literature and legislation, speaking with individuals from the field, and discussing the issue with relevant associations and groups. Depending on the complexity of the issue, experts in the field are consulted and expert panels are convened to discuss the issue further. The Joint Commission reviews the current standards to determine if the problem is new or if the problem is already managed by an existing standard that may need to be revised [11].

Regardless of whether a standard needs to be revised or newly created, certain goals are used as guides in its development. The standards must focus on those functions and aspects of patient care that are essential to the safety and quality of patient care. They must state, whenever possible, the objectives or principles to be met. Rather than specific mechanisms for meeting requirements, they must be reasonable, achievable, and surveyable [12].

Keeping these goals in mind, standards are developed that lead an organization to provide quality care, treatment, and services related to the issue, by defining performance expectations, structures, or processes that need to be put in place. Several standard components are then developed. An introductory text is written that gives information about, and frames, the issue. Background information, justification, or additional information is covered by the new standard's rationale. The actual "to do" items of a standard are the elements of performance, which delineate the need to implement the specific performance expectations, structures, or processes.

The revision or draft of the standard is then reviewed by the relevant Professional and Technical Advisory Committee (PTAC). Each program, be it hospital, ambulatory care, behavioral health, and so forth, has its own PTAC, comprising representatives from professional associations and the public. The standard is then further reviewed by the Standard and Survey Process Committee (SSP), composed of board members, PTAC vice chairs, and at-large members [13]. The SSP resolves concerns raised by the PTAC and gives the final approval for the draft and for a field review of the standard. Depending on the scope of the standard, the field review can be general or specific. Requests to participate are sent out to the field, and draft standards are posted on the Web site. Information based on reaction to the standard and input to specific questions is collected by way of a Web-enabled database. Consultation with advisory groups such as program-specific groups, business groups, or public groups may be performed. An internal review of the input received from all the above sources is made, concerns raised by the field are identified, and changes to the standard draft are made. The standard is then resubmitted for approval by the PTAC and the SSP. The verbiage is finalized, and decisions are made on how compliance will be determined by the surveyors and how the new standard will be placed and integrated into existing standards. The final draft of the standard is then submitted to the Joint Commission Board of Commissioners, which either approves the standard for publication or sends it back for revisions.

Once a standard has been approved by the board of commissioners, surveyors are educated on the new standard and the survey protocols. The field is notified through articles in Joint Commission publications and on the Web site. Finally, the standard is incorporated into the continuous standard review and refinement process, which occurs every 2 years for each of the manuals [11,14].

Standards improvement initiative

In 2006, The Joint Commission launched a massive standards improvement initiative as part of its continuous effort to improve the clarity and relevance of its standards. The goal of the initiative is to eliminate nonessential standards and to ensure that the remaining standards are clearer and more applicable to the care settings at which they are aimed. For example, all compound sentences and bulleted requirements will be eliminated or broken down so that only one specific requirement is addressed. Additionally, the standards manuals will be reorganized to align better with the patient care process and the scoring will be more straightforward. Another welcomed change would be the highlighting of standards that require actual documentation to prove compliance. The hospital program, ambulatory program, office-based surgery programs, critical access hospital program, and home care program have a roll-out target date of January 2009; the other programs will follow.

Following the mantra, "Helping health care organizations help patients," the standards improvement initiative involves extensive communication and interaction with health care organizations to gain their perspectives and advice on how to improve the content and organization of the standards. Feedback is sought from accredited and nonaccredited health care organizations, Joint Commission advisory groups, payers, purchasers, consumers, governmental agencies, experts, and Joint Commission surveyors. Comments and field input are gathered through on-line surveys, meetings, one-on-one interviews, and focus groups [11].

Joint Commission accountability and oversight

Over the years, The Joint Commission has benefited and grown as a result of its acceptance as an accrediting body from the federal government. At the same time, because of governmental oversight and criticism, The Joint Commission has challenged itself to remain an unbiased, voluntary oversight agency. The Hill Burton Act of 1946 was the first time Congress openly validated the value and credibility of the JCAH accreditation process. Another triumph for the JCAH occurred with the Social Security Amendments of 1965. The amendments enabled hospitals accredited by the JCAH to be deemed compliant with Medicare conditions of participation, a practice which continues today [4]. Up until the Medicare Act of 1972, the government did not have a formal policy validating compliancy and accrediting of hospitals by the JCAH. The Ribicoff amendments addressed this and as a result, the US Department of Health, Education and Welfare (HEW) was given the authority to conduct validation surveys on accredited hospitals seeking Medicare reimbursements. The amendments went one step further and authorized HEW to conduct validation surveys when complaints of noncompliance were generated [4]. The JCAH continued to face more scrutiny, but this time, engineers and fire experts from the Bureau of Health Insurance in the Social Security Administration were validating the JCAH's surveys. As a result of these validation surveys, between 1973 and 1975, 105 hospitals lost their deemed status. In response, the JCAH hired more of its own experts to conduct surveys and focused on revising the written standards [4]. The US General Accounting Office (GAO) also began its own in-depth investigations. The GAO's 1979 and 1980s reports were more favorable to the JCAH and, once again, the JCAH was regaining the trust of the public and organizations [4]. The 1990 GAO report was not as favorable; shortcomings were identified [4] because of discrepancies in standard compliance findings. Consistency in evaluation processes to maintain stakeholder confidence is continually being reformulated. Surveyor training occurs annually to ensure the inter-rater reliability of standard compliance evaluation.

Public disclosure and information dissemination

Concurrent with performance improvement initiatives, the JCAHO's continued focus on public awareness took off in 1993. The number of public members on the board increased to six and a nursing representative was added. Over the next 7 years, an organization's survey findings and the number and nature of substantiated complaints filed against it were released to the public for the first time. The JCAHO–accredited organizational performance reports were also released and became available on the JCAHO Web site in 1997 as a part of Quality Check. A huge success, the site boosts 90,000 hits per month. Another consumer-focused initiative was the implementation of a JCAHO toll-free hotline. Patients and their caregivers could now voice their concerns over the care received from accredited health care organizations. The Public Advisory Group on Healthcare Quality was also established. This group's function was to keep the JCAHO abreast of the public's expectations for quality in health care, and to express what health care issues were of public concern [3].

Future of The Joint Commission: improving health outcomes

After leading The Joint Commission for more than 20 years, President Dr. Dennis O'Leary is stepping down. His successor, Mark R. Chassin, MD, MPP, MPH, brings with him a solid foundation of experience in state and federal regulation, research, and risk management. His focus will be on improving health outcomes for patients, specifically "...real and durable...I would like to go beyond measurement and accreditation to facilitate that kind of improvement in quality and safety in accredited organizations...We need more and better measures of quality, ones that address a wider spectrum of health care. In that development process, however, we must never lose sight of the absolute necessity to be as sure as we can that improvement on those measures will translate directly into improved outcomes for patients" [15].

Dr. Chassin insightfully recognizes that organizations are unsure of the best approach to achieve improved outcomes. He envisions the Joint Commission and Joint Commission resources playing a major role in the delivery of tools to aid their quest. "However, I would like to emphasize the need to understand the specific needs of accredited organizations as they initiate improvements and to then respond with high-quality products and services from The Joint Commission and Joint Commission Resources. I want us to take part in the process of creating, in a careful and rigorous way, the necessary tools and metrics and then disseminating them to organizations. We should be able to provide organizations with generalizable lessons so that they save time and resources from developing tools on their own and move more rapidly toward improvement" [15].

Dr. Chassin is keenly aware of the financial burdens and resource constraints organizations face in pursuing improved outcomes. In the following quote he clearly identifies the need to balance these with standards and metrics. "We must have a high level of confidence that the actions that we are asking organizations to take improve patient outcomes. We will be careful to focus on the actions, then, that have the greatest effect on outcomes, and that have a beneficial long-term impact on organizations. We must also be mindful of the opportunity costs in undertaking a given improvement activity, for it takes the organization's resources away from other improvement activities in which it might otherwise be engaged. There is a need to prune this garden to ensure that scarce resources are deployed in the most beneficial interventions" [15].

Summary

Ninety-seven years after the death of Florence Nightingale and sixty-seven years after the death of Dr. Codman, for the first time the government has taken an end-result, outcomes management approach to billing. The August 22, 2007, CMS report announced that, beginning in 2008, the CMS will not reimburse hospitals for the costs of patient care resulting from certain preventable errors, injuries, or infections that could have been reasonably prevented. Equally impressive, the CMS will not reimburse organizations for the care required as a result of serious preventable events. Specifically, the eight conditions included in the report are: retained foreign objects after surgery, air embolism, blood incompatibility, catheter-associated urinary tract infections, decubitus ulcers, vascular-associated infections, surgical site infections, and hospital-acquired injuries [16].

The question of whether or not health care is safer today remains debatable. Certainly, public and professional awareness is at an all-time high. Only with continued outcomes management and evidence-based medicine will health care continue to move toward improved patient safety and optimal patient care. By continuing to focus on the quality management of systems and process issues, organizations will continue to strengthen and build on the foundation of patient safety started by Florence Nightingale.

References

[1] Ulrich B. Leadership and management according to Florence Nightingale. Norwalk (CT): Appleton and Lange; 1992. p. 10.

[2] Mallon WJ. The genesis of the end result. In: Ernest Amory Codman: the end result of a life in medicine. Philadelphia: W.B. Saunders Company; 2000. p. 47–70.

[3] A journey through the history of the joint commission. The Joint Commission Web site. Available at: http://www.jointcommission.org/AboutUs/joint_commission_history.htm. Accessed June 20, 2007.

[4] Brauer CM. Champions of quality in health care. Lyme (CT): Greenwich Publishing Group Inc.; 2001. p. 17, 22, 26, 30, 44, 54, 62, 68, 80, 109.

[5] Mallon WJ. A study in hospital efficiency. In: Ernest Amory Codman: the end result of a life in medicine. Philadelphia: W.B. Saunders Company; 2000. p. 83–94.

[6] Kohn LT, Corrigan JM, Donaldson MS, editors. To err is human, building a safer health system. Washington, DC: National Academy Press; 2000. p. 26, 42.

[7] Mallon WJ. Ernest Amory Codman: the end result of a life in medicine. Philadelphia: W.B. Saunders Company; 2000. p. 92.

[8] A journey through the history of the joint commission. Sentinel events. The Joint Commission Web site. Available at: http://www.jointcommission.org/SentinelEvents/PolicyandProcedures/. Accessed June 20, 2007.

[9] Facts about ORYX® for hospitals, core measures and hospital core measures. The Joint Commission Web site. Available at: http://www.jointcommission.org/AccreditationPrograms/Hospitals/ORYX/Oryx_facts.htm. Accessed October 1, 2007.

[10] Accreditation process. Facts about the tracer methodology. The Joint commission Web site. Available at: http://www.jointcommission.org/AccreditationPrograms/Hospitals/AccreditationProcess/Tracer_Methodology.htm. Accessed August 31, 2007.

[11] Kupka N. Standards development. Presented at: 2003 Annual Invitational Conference. Chicago (IL), January 2003.

[12] Barnett S. The Joint Commission on Accreditation of Healthcare Organizations orientation guide for military fellows 2006–2007. 2006.

[13] Wise R. The development of a standard. Presented at an SSP Committee Meeting. Oakbrook Terrace (IL), 2007.

[14] Dunlap KD, Shell CM. I never knew that...Joint Commission series. Army Nurse Corps Newsletter 2006:2.

[15] An interview with Dr. Mark Chassin, next president of the Joint Commission. The Joint Commission Perspectives 2007;27(10):1–3.

[16] Medicare to eliminate additional payments for certain hospital acquired conditions. Fed Regist 2007;72(162):7129–8175.

ELSEVIER
SAUNDERS

Perioperative Nursing Clinics 3 (2008) 27–33

PERIOPERATIVE
NURSING
CLINICS

Business Plan Mobile Surgical Platform Use in Perioperative Continuum: Staff Injury Reduction

Erin Lawler, MS

Department of Defense Patient Safety Center, 1335 East West Highway, Suite 6-100, Silver Spring, MD 20910, USA

Nursing is a high-risk occupation for work-related musculoskeletal disorders (MSDs), and it continues to rank among the leading occupations with associated lost work time. According to the US Bureau of Labor Statistics, registered nurses ranked eighth in number of work-related MSDs with days away from work in 2005, totaling 9060 reported injuries with a median of 7 missed workdays per injury [1]. Nurses' aides, orderlies, and attendants ranked second behind laborers and freight, stock, and material movers, with 28,920 work-related musculoskeletal injuries and a median of 5 days of missed work (Table 1). Fifty-eight percent of the injuries, which were usually strains and sprains due to overexertion, involved patient handling [1].

Work-related MSDs are not only financially costly to a health care organization, averaging more than $160,000 per 100,000 work hours [2], but can significantly decrease the workforce necessary to deliver health care effectively, efficiently, and safely. Having fewer, or physically compromised, personnel to perform health care duties can have far-reaching implications, such as insufficient staffing levels, greater workloads on other employees, longer shifts, shorter recovery periods between shifts, staff burnout, and greater risk for physical strain [3–5]. Such strained conditions can affect patient safety, increasing the risk of adverse patient outcomes [3,4].

This article is sponsored by the Armed Forces Institute of Pathology, Washington, DC.

The opinions or assertions herein are those of the author and do not necessarily reflect the views of the Department of the Army, Navy, or Air Force or of the Department of Defense.

E-mail address: lawlerl@afip.osd.mil

The objective of enhancing staff safety is critical and action is growing to address the risks of work-related MSDs related to patient handling in health care. The purpose of this article is to identify current patient-handling initiatives, the limitations to implementing these programs successfully, and the need for incorporating preventative design interventions that minimize the overall need for patient handling.

Musculoskeletal disorders in nursing

MSDs often involve the soft tissues of the body, including muscles, ligaments, nerves, tendons, joints, and cartilage [1], and the most common MSD injuries in nursing involve the back, neck, and shoulders. Although many other activities, such as feeding and bathing a patient, can require maintaining awkward postures and can cause strain and overexertion, most MSDs in nursing occur from patient-handling activities characterized by repetitive lifting, turning, repositioning, and laterally transferring patients [6]. A nurse typically lifts 1.8 tons cumulative weight over an 8-hour shift [7,8], and bending over with the trunk flexed has been found to be the most frequent posture for nurses [9]. The highest risk activities include transferring patients to and from toilets, chairs, bathtubs, and beds, and transferring between these surfaces; lifting, repositioning, or turning patients; changing the bed when a patient is in it; and dressing or undressing a patient [6,9,10].

The effects of strains and sprains to the back, neck, and shoulders due to patient handling have been well documented [9,11,12]. One study found that more than one half of the strains and sprain injuries reported for seven northeast hospitals during the 2000 and 2001 calendar year periods were

1556-7931/08/$ - see front matter. Published by Elsevier Inc.
doi:10.1016/j.cpen.2007.11.002

Table 1
Number of work-related musculoskeletal disorders involving days away from work and median days away from work by selected occupations, 2005

	Number	Median days away from work
Total musculoskeletal disorders	375,540	9
Laborers and freight, stock, and material movers, hand	32,100	9
Nursing aides, orderlies, and attendants	28,920	5
Truck drivers, heavy and tractor-trailer	18,330	14
Truck drivers, light or delivery services	11,760	10
Janitors and cleaners, except maids and housekeeping cleaners	10,470	9
Retail salespersons	9800	9
Stock clerks and order fillers	9600	7
Registered nurses	9060	7
Construction laborers	8540	10
Maintenance and repair workers, general	6870	7
Carpenters	6630	10
Maids and housekeeping cleaners	6320	8
First-line supervisors/ managers of retail sales workers	5570	14
Cashiers	5510	8
Automotive service technicians and mechanics	4610	12

From US Department of Labor Bureau of Labor Statistics. Nonfatal occupational injuries and illnesses requiring days away from work. Available at: http://www.bls.gov/iif/home.htm. Accessed September 20, 2007.

related to patient-handling tasks (68.7% and 68.6%, respectively) [13]. Patient-handling tasks accounted for four out of the top five occupational injury–causing activities; repositioning patients was the highest risk task, accounting for 17.9% of reported injuries during the 24-month period. Lifting and transferring patients in and out of a bed or chair were the third- and fourth-leading injury-causing tasks, and lateral patient transfers were the eighth-leading injury-causing task, accounting for 5.7% of reported injuries [13].

These strenuous tasks are exacerbated by multiple challenges unique to health care.

Patient-handling tasks often occur in restrictive environmental conditions, and in awkward and mechanically stressful positions that are sustained over prolonged durations and variable distances [14–18]. Patients also have variable sizes, shapes, and weights, which can impede maintaining neutral and proper biomechanics. In one Department of Veterans Affairs hospital, patients weighed, on average, 169 pounds, with a range of 91 to 387 pounds [17]. Physical and cognitive dependencies, patient behaviors, and levels of cooperation can also vary, which can affect weight distribution and the strength needed to counter awkward patient movement. It has been shown that lateral sheer, anterior-posterior sheer, spine compression, and torso twisting increase in relation to the degree of asymmetry in team lifting tasks, and lateral sheer forces have been shown to approach the tolerance limits within the intervertebral discs [19]. Asymmetric lifting origins and destinations are common for patient-handling tasks, which often occur while bending over or in adverse postures and with lifting teams that are physically mismatched. These variables can increase risks for back injuries or other MSDs.

Perioperative nurses are not only vulnerable to high-risk tasks, such as vertical and lateral patient transfers to or from an operating table, repositioning patients, holding patient extremities for prepping, and moving heavy equipment [20,21] but are exposed to additional risks related to static loading of soft tissues during procedures, which can exacerbate existing injuries and increase the potential for injury from overexerting already fatigued muscles and strained tendons [22,23]. Prolonged standing, lifting and pushing equipment, maintaining awkward postures, holding retractors for prolonged periods, reaching, and adverse environmental conditions have been identified as the leading injury-causing categories for operating room personnel [24].

Given the work demands and conditions, nurses and caregivers are particularly vulnerable to back injuries. One study found that 65% of operating room nurses and 58% of intensive care nurses had had at least one work-related low back injury throughout their career and roughly three quarters of reported incidences of current MSDs were for low back pain [9]. Another study found 47% of 1163 working nurses had had a back MSD during the last year [12].

As a result, nursing injuries are among the costliest in terms of lost workdays and worker's compensation claims [2,14,25], and health care–related back injury claims lead back-related compensatory claims among industries [22]. Back injuries among nurses have been found to have an annual prevalence of 40% to 50% and a lifetime prevalence of 35% to 80% [26], and estimates indicate that 12% to 18% transfer out of nursing personnel jobs because of chronic back pain [15]. Indirect costs, such as work interruption and worker replacement and training, have been estimated to be between two and five times direct injury costs [13,27]. Costs of work-related MSDs become salient and more critical when considering the increasing obesity rates, which present unique health care needs requiring additional equipment and staffing resources [28]. Other considerations include the growing nursing shortage [27], which may lead to longer work hours and more responsibilities for personnel, creating further risks for MSDs [29], and the estimated aging of nursing personnel, whose current average age is in the mid-forties. Muscle strength decreases with age, leading to higher risk for low back pain and injury [13].

It is, thus, critical that manual patient lifting be minimized or eliminated, and that technologic innovations be introduced in patient care settings that eliminate the need for moving and transferring patients and give ergonomic mechanical advantage when patient movement must be performed.

Biomechanical effects of patient handling and movement

Patient lifting, repositioning, and lateral transfers have been shown to increase spinal loading and cause back strain. Injuries can occur from isolated overexertion and from the cumulative effects of repeatedly performing the high-risk activities associated with preparing a patient for mechanical transfer. Traditional ways of addressing high-risk activities and vulnerabilities to work-related MSDs, such as incorporating proper biomechanics training and education on proper lifting techniques, have proved ineffective for reducing back injuries and musculoskeletal strain related to patient handling [14,26,30,31]. Given the overwhelming direct and indirect costs of work-related musculoskeletal injuries, momentum is growing to embrace no-lift or safe patient-handling initiatives, as reflected in the Association of periOperative Registered Nurses (AORN) position statement, which states that "AORN is committed to the attainment and maintenance of an ergonomically healthy workplace to protect all employees in the perioperative setting" [22] and calls for the availability of assistive patient-handling equipment and the development of policies regarding manual patient handling. The most common mechanical devices include either ceiling-mounted or portable full-body slings to transfer dependent patients; stand-assist devices to transfer partially dependent, weight-bearing patients; and lateral transfer devices, such as sliding boards or inflatable mattresses, for transferring between lateral surfaces [17,32].

The efficacy of using mechanical ceiling lifts, stand-assist lifts, and other assistive devices is well documented and they show reductions in MSDs, back injuries, and perceived risk of injury and exertion, and increases in cost savings due to reductions in compensation claims and lost work, and personnel satisfaction [14,32–40]. The most successful programs are multilayered initiatives that support administrative, engineering, and behavioral controls where personnel are trained in how to use the devices, have immediate access to equipment and lifting teams, and have policies to dictate and support when and how to move patients [14,30,31,34].

However, despite the advantages of mechanical lifting devices for reducing peak compressive forces on the spine and surrounding back muscles [41,42], evidence suggests that the activities involved in preparing a person for a mechanical lift or transfer, such as rotating a patient from side to side, lifting the torso or legs, or bending over for a long duration, can have equally harmful cumulative effects [17,35]. Spinal compressive and sheer forces can mount during a patient-handling incident, over the duration of a work shift, and from exposure throughout a worker's lifetime. The accumulation of the stressors over time can have harmful effects, particularly for tasks that are repeated frequently during a shift. Although peak compression loads decreased when using assistive devices during five common patient-handling activities, such as bed-to-wheelchair transfers, repositioning, and bed-to-stretcher transfers, cumulative sheer reaction forces and spinal loading were shown to increase when using assistive devices in one study. It was concluded that the forces increased because of prolonged time spent bent forward in flexed positions to prepare a patient for movement [35]. Time to perform the patient-movement task was significantly greater than manual tasks, leading to more time spent in awkward positions.

The actions involved in preparing for manual or mechanical transfers can take time to complete, and each individual action can impose different biomechanical stressors on the body. Zhuang and colleagues [43] (1999) measured the effects of six transfer methods on the biomechanical stress of nursing personnel involved in patient handling. Stand-up powered lifts, an overhead lift, basket sling lifts, a sliding board, a walking belt, and no assistive devices (manual) were compared using two elderly patients as residents. Back compressive forces were highest, with an average 3487 N, during the two-person baseline manual transfer task of lifting the patient's torso and rotating the patient to the side of the bed in preparation for standing. Lifting the legs produced a 3157 N average back compressive force. One-person tasks of rotating patients to prepare for either slide board transfers or stand-up lifts produced an average 3454 N compressive force, whereas rolling patients toward and away from the nurse produced the lowest compressive forces of 2951 N and 2698 N, respectively. Despite using assistive devices, many of the mean compressive forces exceeded the National Institute for Occupational Safety and Health (NIOSH) back-compression criterion limit of 3400 N when preparing to use the device, and this does not take into account the cumulative load effects of sustaining awkward positions for periods of time. Mean compressive forces increased when moving a heavier patient and this was also true for hand forces required to move the patient [43].

Push, pull, and rotate forces can also vary among mechanical lift devices, with floor-based assistive lifts requiring higher forces than ceiling lifts to move and position a patient properly, which may increase the cumulative loading effects on the back, shoulders, arms, and knees [17,44]. One study found that floor-based lifts required seven times more rotation force to move a patient and reported that people with smaller frames, such as women, would not have the necessary strength to perform specific patient-handling tasks with a fully loaded lift [44].

Patient transfers between lateral surfaces, such as from a stretcher to an operating table or from a bed to a stretcher, also place considerable strain on the back, arms, and shoulders [16,17,45]. Because of the biomechanically awkward positions and extended reach required to pull a draw sheet, and the increasing forces required to move heavier patients, transferring patients between lateral surfaces is one of the highest risk patient-handling

activities, increasing sheer forces on the lateral and anterior-posterior planes [15,34,46]. Assistive devices, such as inflatable mattresses, friction-reducing devices, and roller boards, have been shown to reduce the sheer and compressive forces to the spine and the shoulder strength required in lateral transfers as compared with manual methods, with moderate-to-limited evidence in support of their use [46–48]. Mechanical devices, such as using an air-assisted transfer device or using mechanical belts, have been shown to require fewer personnel to operate (two people versus three people for manual devices) and were perceived to require less physical exertion, and patients reported an increased sense of security and comfort when transferred using mechanical assistive devices over that of sliding boards or draw sheets [27].

Despite the availability of mechanical transfer devices, manual methods, including sliding boards and draw sheets, continue to be the most pervasive assistive devices [27] with draw sheets the most popular method [34]. However, draw sheets have been shown to cause sheer anterior-posterior strain on the intervertebral discs [34], require an applied force of 646 N to push or pull a patient [16], and are not as effective in reducing spinal forces [31]. Manual methods have been shown to create compressive forces on L5/S1 discs well above the NIOSH–recommended back compression limit of 3400 N [49]. Friction-reducing devices like slide boards still require the force and strength to move a patient manually, which can increase cumulative load effects [16], and the forces required to move a patient increase as a function of weight, despite using friction-reducing devices [45,46]. One study found that nurses with slide boards and draw sheets available were more likely to have a back MSD compared with nurses who had lifting teams and devices readily available [31].

Limitations of mechanical assistive devices

Despite the biomechanical stresses patient-handling devices can impart on the body, mechanical lifting and transfer devices have been shown to reduce the risks of MSDs and injuries to the back effectively, compared with manual lifting and transfer methods, and have proved to be safer for nurses and patients.

However, several limitations counter the usefulness and frequency of use of these devices. Nurses have been shown to have negative views of patient-handling devices [20,50]. The most common reasons for not using the devices are increased time to operate; lack of need to perform patient-handling task; instability and safety issues; inaccessible or unavailable equipment; inability to locate equipment; perceived patient discomfort; maneuverability and space restrictions; lack of a standardized patient safety policy; insufficient training; difficulty in operating; unintuitive functions; and poor maintenance (see Refs. [15,17,20,34,35,41]).

Several studies noted a lack of compliance in using mechanical lifting devices, even when such equipment was available, despite the high risks of acquiring a back injury or other MSDs [26,39]. In one study, manual assistive devices, such as sliding boards and draw sheets, were used more often than mechanical assistive devices, such as sit-stand and sling lifts, despite the latter's availability [9]. Trinkoff and colleagues [31] found that using mechanical lifting devices ranked third behind two-person lifts and a lifting team as the most preferred method of patient handling.

Device use has also been found to vary by care specialty, with lift teams being the preferred patient-handling method for oncology nurses and postanesthesia units, for example [31]. Use has been shown to vary by care facility (with significantly higher use in a long-term care facility as opposed to an acute care facility) and by staff (registered nurses used mechanical lifts less frequently than other nursing personnel) [39]. Compliance has also been shown to vary according to transfer task and patient weight, with compliance increasing with greater patient weights and subsequent perceived risk [35].

Concerted attention should be given to addressing the limitations of using patient lifts and other assistive devices. The noted user behaviors, reported opinions, and inconsistency in using assistive devices provide valuable evidence that more action is needed to ensure that safe patient-handling programs, technology, and work design efficiently and effectively support the abilities and needs of the caregiver. The patient-handling movement would benefit from not only continued evidence-based research in establishing more cost-effective, efficient, and accessible patient movement devices but also research into design interventions that address minimizing the need for using assistive devices.

Mobile surgical table as an engineering control

A need will always exist to move or reposition patient limbs and to lift patients from the bed to a chair, or chair to bathtub or toilet, and so forth, and mechanical assistive devices should be used during these activities when the condition of the patient allows for it. However, it has been shown that the body will endure some strain and stress even when using mechanical lift devices, and, over time, the cumulative effect may lead to MSDs. The NIOSH lifting parameters set forth in 1993, which include a minimum horizontal lifting distance and a maximum weight to be lifted of 51 lbs under ideal conditions, and which are used in many of these studies, are considered inapplicable given the unique, often unpredictable lifting conditions and tasks of nursing care [18,34,44]. Revised NIOSH parameters for patient handling identify 35 lbs as the maximum weight to be lifted under ideal circumstances, and less for lifting in awkward positions (squatting, twisting, arms extended, and so forth), for lifting in constrictive spaces, or for working more than 8 hours [18]. Most patient-handling tasks, therefore, put a person at considerable risk of injury according to the new parameters, which can be exacerbated by the repetitive movement and continual strain often experienced during a shift. Reducing the frequency with which caregivers have to move a patient manually, including in preparation to use a mechanical device, is as critical as the need to reduce the physical strain and exertion experienced during these activities.

Design interventions that eliminate the need for patient handling would be an essential component to the current patient-handling programs of administrative no-lift policies, mechanical lifting and transfer devices, and effective training. Innovative patient bed designs exist in which beds are equipped with assistive patient repositioning features, or they convert to chairs, eliminating high-risk bed-to-chair and chair-to-bed patient-handling tasks (see Refs. [15,17,26,32,34]). Yet lateral transfers would still occur among operating room tables, stretchers, and patient beds. Although some patient movement and repositioning tasks are necessary and unavoidable, some lateral transfers are not intrinsically essential and could be reduced or eliminated with thoughtful design. An engineering control of designing one bed to function for multiple lateral surface needs (stretcher, operating room table, patient bed) throughout a patient's care lifecycle could eliminate the need for some lateral transfers, further preventing risks for MSDs related to this high-risk activity. Design solutions like this help to address the fundamental issue of eliminating unnecessary patient movement, which could, in turn, reduce the overall volume of patient movement tasks, increase the accessibility of assistive devices for other patient-handling needs, and reduce the risks of injury to patients during transfer.

Opportunities to integrate innovative, safe patient-handling technologies throughout the patient care cycle abound. As the patient safety movement evolves, more evidence-based research is needed with respect to design interventions that minimize patient handling, particularly in measuring the effect multifunctional beds might have on reducing MSDs among caregivers. Although mobile operating room tables may not be a panacea in terms of eliminating the need for caregivers to rotate patients and reposition limbs, multifunctional beds used holistically with assistive devices, training, and administrative controls may be a significant addition to the safe patient-handling toolkit.

References

[1] U.S Department of Labor Bureau of Labor Statistics. Nonfatal occupational injuries and illnesses requiring days away from work. 2005:1–31. Available at: http://www.bls.gov/iif/home.htm. Accessed September 20, 2007.

[2] Siddharthan K, Nelson A, Weisenbom G. A business case for patient care ergonomic interventions. Nurs Adm Q 2005;29(1):63–71.

[3] Hall LM, Doran D, Pink G. Nurse staffing models, nursing hours, and patient safety outcomes. J Nurs Adm 2004;34(1):41–5.

[4] Aiken LH, Clarke SP, Sloane DM, et al. Hospital nurse staffing and patient mortality, nurse burnout, and job dissatisfaction. JAMA 2002;288(16):1987–93.

[5] Rogers AE, Hwang WT, Scott LD, et al. The working hours of hospital staff nurses and patient safety. Health Aff 2004;23(4):203–12.

[6] Owen B, Garg A. Reducing risk for back pain in nursing personnel. AAOHN J 1991;39:24–33.

[7] Touhy-Main K. Why manual handling should be eliminated for resident and career safety. Geriaction 1997;15:10–4.

[8] Retsas A, Pinikahana J. Manual handling activities and injuries among nurses: an Australian hospital study. J Adv Nurs 2000;31:875–83.

[9] Viera ER, Kumar S, Coury HJCG, et al. Low back problems and possible improvements in nursing jobs. Journal of Advanced Nursing 2006;55(1):79–89.

[10] Menzel NN, Brooks ST, Bernard TE, et al. The physical workload of nursing personnel: association with musculoskeletal discomfort. Int J Nurs Stud 2004;41:859–67.

[11] Marras WS, Davis KG, Kirking BC, et al. A comprehensive analysis of low-back disorder risk and spinal loading during the transferring and repositioning of patients using different techniques-Ergonomics 1999;42(7):904–26.

[12] Trinkoff AM, Lipscomb JA, Geiger-Brown J, et al. Musculoskeletal problems of the neck, shoulder, and back and functional consequences in nurses. Am J Ind Med 2002;41:170–8.

[13] Fragala G, Bailey LB. Addressing sprains and strains: musculoskeletal injuries in hospitals. AAOHN J 2003;51(6):252–9.

[14] Nelson A, Matz M, Chen F, et al. Development and evaluation of a multifaceted ergonomics program to prevent injuries associated with patient handling tasks. Int J Nurs Stud 2006;43:717–33.

[15] Nelson A, Baptiste AS. Evidence-based practices for safe patient handling and movement. Orthop Nurs 2006;25(6):366–79.

[16] Lloyd JD, Baptiste A. Friction-reducing devices for lateral patient transfers: a biomechanical evaluation. AAOHN J 2006;54(3):113–9.

[17] Nelson A, Fragala G, Menzel N. Myths and facts about back injuries in nursing. Am J Nurs 2003; 103(2):32–40.

[18] Waters TR. When is it safe to manually lift a patient? The revised NIOSH lifting equation provides support for recommended weight limits. Am J Nurs 2007;107(8):53–8.

[19] Marras WS, Davis KG, Kirking BC, et al. Spine loading and trunk kinematics during team lifting. Ergonomics 1999;42(10):1258–73.

[20] Owen B. Preventing injuries using an ergonomic approach. AORN J 2000;72(6):1031–6.

[21] Wicker P. Manual handling in the perioperative environment. Br J Perioper Nurs 2000;10(5):255–9.

[22] Proposed position statements. Ergonomically healthy workplace practices. AORN J 2006;83(1):119–22.

[23] Sparkman CAG. Ergonomics in the workplace. AORN J 2006;84(3):379–82.

[24] Meijsen P, Knibbe HJJ. Work-related musculoskeletal disorders of perioperative personnel in The Netherlands. AORN J 2007;86(2):193–208.

[25] de Castro AB. Actively preventing injury: avoiding back injuries and other musculoskeletal disorders among nurses. Am J Nurs 2004;104(1):104.

[26] Hignett S. Work-related back pain in nurses. J Adv Nurs 1996;23(6):1238–46.

[27] Pellino TA, Owen B, Knapp L, et al. The evaluation of mechanical devices for lateral transfers on perceived exertion and patient comfort. Orthop Nurs 2006;25(1):4–10.

[28] Dybec RB. Intraoperative positioning and care for the obese patient. Plast Surg Nurs 2004;24(3):118–22.

[29] Lipscomb JA, Trinkoff AM, Geiger-Brown, et al. Work-schedule characteristics and reported musculoskeletal disorders of registered nurses. Scand J Work Environ Health 2002;28(6):394–401.

[30] Hignett S. Intervention strategies to reduce musculo-skeletal injuries associated with handling patients: a systematic review. Occup Environ Med 2003; 60(6):1–8. Available at: http//:www.oem.bmj.com. Accessed August 30, 2007.

[31] Trinkoff AM, Brady B, Nielsen K. Workplace prevention and musculoskeletal injuries in nurses. J Nurs Adm 2003;33(3):153–8.

[32] Nelson A, Owen B, Lloyd JD, et al. Safe patient handling and movement. Am J Nurs 2003;103(3): 32–43.

[33] Owen B, Keene K, Olson S. An ergonomic approach to reducing back/shoulder stress in hospital nursing personnel: a five year follow up. Int J Nurs Stud 2002;39:295–302.

[34] Nelson A, Lloyd JD, Menzel N, et al. Preventing nursing back injuries: redesigning patient handling tasks. AAOHN J 2003;51(3):126–34.

[35] Daynard D, Yassi A, Cooper JE, et al. Biomechanical analysis of peak and cumulative spinal loads during simulated patient-handling activities: a substudy of a randomized controlled trial to prevent lift and transfer injury of health care workers. Appl Ergon 2001;32:199–214.

[36] Yassi A, Cooper JE, Tate RB, et al. A randomized controlled trial to prevent patient lift and transfer injuries of health care workers. Spine 2001;26(16): 1739–46.

[37] Li J, Wolf L, Evanoff B. Use of mechanical patient lifts decreased musculoskeletal symptoms and injuries among health care workers. Inj Prev 2004; 10:212–6. Available at: http://www.injury.prevention.bmj.com. Accessed September 19, 2007.

[38] Engst C, Chhokar R, Miller A, et al. Effectiveness of overhead lifting devices in reducing the risk of injury to care staff in extended care facilities. Ergonomics 2005;48(2):187–99.

[39] Evanoff B, Wolf L, Aton E, et al. Reduction in injury rates in nursing personnel through introduction of mechanical lifts in the workplace. Am J Ind Med 2003;44:451–7.

[40] Miller A, Engst C, Tate RB, et al. Evaluation of the effectiveness of portable ceiling lifts in a new long-term care facility. Appl Ergon 2006;37:377–85.

[41] Keir PJ, MacDonell CW. Muscle activity during patient transfers: a preliminary study on the influence of lift assists and experience. Ergonomics 2004;47(3):296–306.

[42] Silvia CE, Bloswick DS, Lillquist D, et al. An ergonomic comparison between mechanical and manual patient transfer techniques. Work 2002;19:19–34.

[43] Zhuang Z, Stobbe TJ, Hsiao H, et al. Biomechanical evaluation of assistive devices for transferring residents. Appl Ergon 1999;30:285–94.

[44] Waters T, Collins J, Galinsky T, et al. NIOSH research efforts to prevent musculoskeletal disorders in the healthcare industry. Orthop Nurs 2006;25(6): 380–9.

[45] Baptiste A, Tiesman H, Nelson A, et al. Technology to reduce nursing back injuries. Rehabil Nurs 2002. Available at: http://www.dergonomics.com. Accessed September 21, 2007.

[46] Bohannan RW. Horizontal transfers between adjacent surfaces: forces required using different methods. Arch Phys Med Rehabil 1999;80:851–3.

[47] Hignett S. Systematic review of patient handling activities starting in lying, sitting and standing positions. J Adv Nurs 2003;41(6):545–52.

[48] Grevelding P, Bohannon RW. Reduced push forces accompany device use during sliding transfers of seated subjects. J Rehabil Res Dev 2001;38(1):135–9.

[49] Ulin SS, Chaffin DB, Patellos CL, et al. Biomechanical analysis of methods used for transferring totally dependent patients. SCI Nurs 1997;14(1):19–27.

[50] Pain H, Jackson S, McLellan DL, et al. User evaluation of handling equipment for moving dependent people in bed. Technology and Disability 1999;11: 13–9.

PERIOPERATIVE
NURSING
CLINICS

Perioperative Nursing Clinics 3 (2008) 35–42

Perioperative Patient Movement: Defining the Issues

George F. Nussbaum, PhD, RN, CNOR

Graduate School of Nursing, Perioperative Clinical Nurse Specialist Program,
Uniformed Services University, 4301 Jones Bridge Road,
Bethesda, MD 20814, USA

Customary business and clinical practice

Conservatively, more than 200,000 surgical procedures are performed daily in surgical treatment facilities in the United States. Not included in this statistic are patients receiving conscious sedation for gastrointestinal, liver, pulmonary, in vitro fertilization, electro-convulsive therapy, and ear, nose, and throat (ENT) procedures performed outside the operating room (OR) [1].

Patients typically begin their surgical procedure process on a patient gurney in a preoperative staging area and are then transferred to an OR and moved onto a standard OR table. At the completion of the surgical procedure, the patient is manually lifted by a minimum of four or more personnel, then laterally transferred to a standard postanesthesia recovery bed and transported to the postanesthesia care unit (PACU). Following phase I recovery in the PACU, the patient is again manually transferred, to a phase II recovery area, an ICU, or an inpatient hospital bed. Each transfer requires a sufficient number of personnel to provide a safe transfer from one platform to another.

A typical surgical patient occupies three to four different transfer or procedural devices, including a gurney, OR table, recovery bed, inpatient or intensive care bed, or a lounge chair prior to discharge. In each instance, the transport or procedure vehicles must be obtained from the storage location where they are awaiting use, cleaned, with fresh bed linen applied, and maintained by medical maintenance personnel. During each transfer, patients are generally inconvenienced, subjected to some degree of risk for falls or related injury,

and must transfer enough of their own body heat to sufficiently warm the device to which they are being transferred. For each patient transfer, a sufficient number of able and available personnel must cease any other activities to attend to the process of safely moving a patient from one device to another (Fig. 1).

The current practice of patient movement through the surgical environment involves significant safety issues for patients and perioperative staff members:

- A sufficient number of personnel must be available to lift and laterally transfer surgical patients from one surface to another, without disrupting vascular access lines, chest tubes, and other drains. Having the appropriate assist devices allows a smooth transfer, provides a minimum of added patient discomfort, and lessens the potentially increased risk for nausea and vomiting during or following movement.
- More than 37% of all staff injuries in hospitals are caused by patient handling and transfer [2]. Federal Employee's Compensation Act (FECA) data from two large teaching facilities, one on the East Coast, the other in the Midwest, the total amount in claims for all back injuries exceeded 2 million dollars for each facility. These dollar amounts do not include paid time off from work or the cost to pay for back-fill personnel. Not all the back injuries occurred exclusively in the perioperative area.
- Avoiding musculoskeletal injuries among perioperative personnel is essential. Transferring patients is only one aspect of the issue. Positioning, holding extremities during

E-mail address: nussbaumgf@verizon.net

1556-7931/08/$ - see front matter © 2008 Elsevier Inc. All rights reserved.
doi:10.1016/j.cpen.2007.11.003

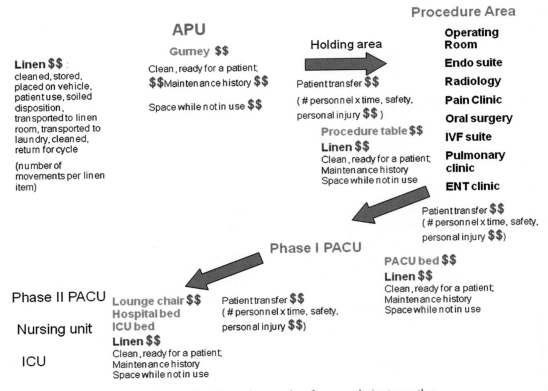

Fig. 1. Process of safely moving a patient from one device to another.

prepping, and lifting large instrument sets are among the other activities that add to the cumulative musculoskeletal trauma of OR nurses. Any effort to reduce the need to lift patients manually should be seriously considered in designing future work-flow processes. A more detailed description and analysis of nursing staff injuries is provided by Lawler elsewhere in this issue.

- Hospital occupancy codes mandate that an 8-foot–clear corridor must be maintained at all times. Fire and safety hazards result when transfer vehicles are located in heavy-traffic patient care areas. To be in compliance with these regulations, one must obtain gurneys and PACU beds from a storage space away from the OR.

Business practice issues include

- Inefficient use of staff time for multiple transfer requirements
- Inefficient use of material resources, including hospital linens, blankets, warming devices, cleaning supplies, and housekeeping personnel

- Inefficient surgical room turnover time
- Inefficient space utilization for transport and recovery vehicles

Recent experiences in specific surgical practices have illustrated the benefits for patients and staff in using a single vehicle for the full spectrum of service of ophthalmology, plastic, and ENT procedures. However, these devices are specific to a limited range of clinical specialties. Traditional OR tables currently used in surgery suites are adaptable for all surgical procedures; however, they are too heavy and impractical to use in a preoperative or postoperative environment. The current use of an OR table necessitates at least two additional vehicles for all procedures performed in surgery.

The transport and treatment modality devices are standard equipment in the surgical environment. The specific purpose, necessity, and added value for each separate vehicle had not been considered or challenged until recently. For more than a decade, adult patients having ophthalmology procedures have been accommodated in special eye surgery beds that effectively eliminate the need for physically lifting and moving a patient from one device to another. The entire surgery and recovery experience became seamless for this surgical subspecialty population on a specifically designed surgery/recovery bed. Several well-known surgical equipment and table manufacturing companies supply these vehicles (Table 1).

Other ambulatory surgical specialty facilities have adapted their practices to a single transport and procedure vehicle to a limited degree, for plastic surgery and ENT procedures. Most of these vehicles are limited to a narrow range of procedures.

Surgical table requirements

A surgical table must support the anesthesia staff and the surgical team's requirements to perform the intended procedures safely for any patient and surgical specialty. These requirements include

- Safe, appropriate access to the surgical site
- Ability to monitor necessary physiologic parameters
- Capability of using C-arm or other imaging modalities during the procedure
- Ability to accommodate necessary positioning devices across a wide range of surgical specialties
- Patient weight capacity adaptable to most of the client population
- Safe pressure management for most procedures
- Simple and reliable functionality
- Ability to adjust to meet the surgeon's physical needs and access to the surgical site
- Facilitation of decrease in surgical room turnover time [3]

Additional specifications should include

- Reducing the number of patient lateral transfers from one platform to another
- Lessening the risk for being a contributing factor in causing perioperative hypothermia

Operating room of the future

The "OR of the Future" (ORF) project began as a research effort to improve work flow efficiencies in the OR and to relieve congestion in the PACU. The research was initiated in the Center for Integration of Medicine and Innovative

Table 1
Representative sample of devices intended for use in preoperative, intraoperative, and postoperative phases of the perioperative procedure

Manufacturer	Model	Surgical specialties supported
TransMotion Medical	TMM5 Surgical Stretcher Chair	Ophthalmology ENT Plastic surgery Outpatient surgery
Midmark	547	Ophthalmology ENT Plastic surgery Dermatology Emergency medicine General surgery
Pedigo	547SLS	Ophthalmology ENT Plastic surgery Dermatology Emergency medicine General surgery
Hill-Rom	TranStar Surgical Stretcher	Ophthalmology ENT Plastic surgery Outpatient/same-day surgery
Steris/Hausted	SurgiStretcher 578-EYE-ST	Ophthalmology ENT Plastic surgery Outpatient/same-day surgery
MAQUET	Operating table system ALPHAMAQUET 1150.30	Ophthalmology ENT Plastic surgery
MAQUET	Operating table system ALPHAMAQUET 1150.19	Gynecology Urology
MAQUET	Operating table system ALPHAMAQUET 1150.23	Urology Vascular surgery Orthopedics
Stryker	Trio Mobile Surgery Platform	Ophthalmology ENT Plastic surgery Gynecology Urology Vascular surgery Orthopedics Pediatrics

Technology and was constructed as a renovation effort at the Massachusetts General Hospital in Boston. The experimental OR is designed and constructed for the purpose of developing, implementing, and assessing the impact of perioperative system changes on OR function [4]. An expressed intent of this research is to create a process efficiency in the nonoperative period [5]. Equipment in the ORF was specifically selected to facilitate patient throughput and to improve efficiencies for surgeons, anesthesia providers, and OR personnel. One method of reducing nonoperative time is to develop new technologies or to modify existing technologies that reduce the time required to accomplish nonoperative tasks. Mobile, exchangeable OR table tops that allow a patient to be transported to and from the OR are examples of such technology. The OR table used in the ORF is a transporter/OR tabletop/fixed column system (MAQUET, Rastatt, Germany) that eliminates OR table-to-gurney surface-to-surface transfers in the OR, which facilitates the rapid transfer of patients between locations [5]. Transporting patients on the operating surface eliminates the need to transfer a patient from one surface to another before and after surgery [6]. Eliminating the need for personnel to lift and laterally transfer patients physically provides the opportunity for parallel processing of work effort, allowing staff to perform other activities prior to patient departure time by reducing patient intraoperative flow time and staff waiting time [7].

Single platform advantages

A single surgical platform allows all patients to begin their surgical procedure in a preoperative area and to remain on the same vehicle from admission to discharge, never having to be moved physically from one device to another by hospital personnel.

The significance for patients and staff in incorporating a single equipment device suitable to use throughout the medical/surgical process is that it may impact

- The frequency of high-risk injury tasks occurring with lateral patient movements on acute and cumulative trauma musculoskeletal spine injuries. Lifting, transferring, and positioning patients areleading causes of fatigue and musculoskeletal pain. Recent biomedical research illustrates that the value of effective manual techniques may be limited. These results indicate the forces exerted on the musculoskeletal system when nurses lift and laterally transfer patients from one platform to another exceed reasonable limits, regardless of techniques used to perform the task [2]. The reduction or elimination of musculoskeletal back injuries resulting from acute or cumulative repetitive patient lifting in procedure areas reduces FECA costs, the loss of personnel due to sick leave, and the costs associated with replacing these workers while on injury status.

- Space requirements. Transport gurneys, OR tables, PACU beds, and ICU beds require a physical space location in the immediate vicinity of the procedure area. Space requirements for multiple transport and procedure vehicles need to be considered for new and OR renovation projects. This space is often an alcove in the hall in the surgery department. Constructing these alcoves for each of the surgical suites usually affects the ultimate size of the OR. Current construction costs for specialty areas such as radiology, labor and delivery, and surgery suites exceed $600 per square foot and are escalating at an annual rate of 18.5% [8]. Reducing the overall square footage required to store and hold empty gurneys and beds awaiting use in recovery areas and surgical areas has a significant impact on construction costs for these critical areas.

- The amount of hospital bed linen required for multiple devices. Each time a patient vacates a transport or procedural platform, the entire vehicle requires terminal cleaning and fresh, clean linens applied. The use of a single platform potentially reduces the amount of linen required and the manpower to transport, store, launder, and replace it.

- Personnel requirements needed for each patient movement from one vehicle to another [7]

- Housekeeping personnel and supplies following utilization of multiple transport/procedure vehicles

- Thermal regulation equipment and materials for each stage of the patient experience, from preprocedure, procedure, postprocedure, to discharge

- Recovery time [9]

- Biomedical support requirements in maintaining a single platform rather than the current multiple inventories of gurneys, procedure tables, and recovery vehicles. Each item of medical equipment requires technical manuals, an inventory of replacement parts, preventive and repair maintenance, and life cycle replacement.

- Throughput time requirements for overall patient procedure encounters [6]
- OR turnover times. Many room cleanup activities can begin prior to the patient leaving the OR because the staff are not waiting to transfer the patient from surface to surface.
- Fire safety hazard violations from gurneys and PACU beds in OR hallways
- Range of clinical procedures that may be performed using a single transport device for ENT, gastrointestinal, pulmonary, plastic, oral, orthopedic, cardiothoracic, and general surgery; neurosurgery; ophthalmology; urology; gynecology; cesarean section; pain clinic; emergency room trauma; electroconvulsive therapy; in vitro fertilization; and bariatric and polytrauma procedures
- Infection control epidemiology issues relating to ability to clean these specific surgical vehicles more thoroughly [10]
- Overall patient and staff satisfaction

Hypothermia

Unintended, nontherapeutic perioperative hypothermia is well documented in past and current medical and nursing literature as a significant issue for all patients undergoing any surgical procedure. Hypothermia is a common experience for most perioperative patients [9,11]. This unpleasant phenomenon starts when a patient undresses and is placed on the initial transport gurney in the preoperative environment, which is the first impression of the caring environment the patient experiences; however, it is usually not the last with respect to thermal comfort and an overall satisfaction with the surgical care. In a survey conducted by Wilson and Kolcaba in 2003 at the American Society of PeriAnesthesia Nurses and the Association of periOperative Registered Nurses conferences, nurses reported thermal comfort as the leading concern for perioperative patients [12,13]. Hypothermia remains an ongoing concern in the full perioperative spectrum, despite the availability of technology to prevent or reduce it [14].

Normal temperature for most patients is in the range of 37°C (98.6°F), whereas the natural state of the gurney platform corresponds with the temperature of the environment, which is a difference of 16° to 20°F between the patient and the transport vehicle. Each time a patient is transferred from one platform to another, as in the case of the gurney to the OR table, and the OR table to a PACU bed, the patient is subjected to a contact temperature that is much lower than normal body temperature, unless surface warming devices are standard for these platforms. A single published article included "lying on cold OR beds" as a contributing factor in the development of hypothermia [15]. In the first hour of the surgical event, a typical patient is moved onto two separate cold surfaces, has the operative site exposed to a cold environment, and prep fluids that eventually evaporate. The thermal insult of vasodilating anesthetic agents, the inhalation of cold volatile gases, and intravenous fluids at room temperature contribute to the overall cooling effect and the resultant hypothermia condition [16].

A patient's core temperature is defined as the temperature of the blood in the central circulatory system. Core temperature measurements can be obtained reliably in the pulmonary artery, esophagus, or tympanic membrane. The threshold between normal and hypothermia is defined by most researchers to be a core temperature less than 96.8°F (36°C) [14,17]. Mild hypothermia refers to core temperatures between 93.2° and 96.8°F (34°–36°C). The balance between heat loss and heat production determines the mean body and core temperatures.

Risk variables that contribute to perioperative hypothermia include

- Age. It is more difficult to prevent hypothermia in older patients and the very young [9,12,13].
- Type of anesthesia. General anesthesia appears to contribute the most to the occurrence of perioperative hypothermia. All inhaled and intravenous anesthetic agents impair thermoregulatory control markedly, by as much as a 0.9 to 2.7°F (1–1.5°C) reduction in core body temperature in the first hour following anesthesia induction [16]. Although hypothermia does occur frequently during regional anesthesia, these procedures are often shorter in duration and the patient may be awake enough to request warming support [9,14,16,18].
- Body fat. Body fat acts as a protective layer. Patients who have a higher percentage of body fat are considered to be less at risk for hypothermia, at least from environmental

variables such as room temperature and surface temperatures of gurneys and OR tables [9].

- Pre-existing conditions. Hypothermia occurs more frequently in patients who have American Society of Anesthesiologists physical status of three or above and endocrine diseases [9].
- Type of surgical procedure (body cavity versus an extremity). Patients having open cavity procedures are at greater risk for hypothermia because of exposed surface and irrigation fluids [16].
- Duration of the procedure. The threat of hypothermia is often underestimated in patients having low-severity and short-duration procedures (less than 1 hour). Patient temperatures are frequently not monitored for relatively minor or routine procedures and patients are often not provided thermal support through nursing interventions sufficient to deter the discomfort of feeling cold [12,16].
- Cold fluid infusion in the forms of IV fluids and irrigation solutions [14].

Hypothermia may include the following adverse economic and physiologic outcomes:

- Mild hypothermia has shown to cause an increased length of PACU stay by decreasing the speed at which the body can metabolize anesthetic agents. Normothermic patients emerge from anesthesia more quickly than hypothermic patients [12,18]. One study determined that patients arriving in the PACU in a mild hypothermic state required approximately 40 to 90 additional minutes in the PACU to reach discharge criteria on the postanesthetic Aldrete and Kroulik recovery scores [9,18].
- Shivering is an involuntary muscular activity that augments metabolic heat production. "Vigorous shivering increases metabolic heat production up to 600% above basal level" [9,19]. Shivering and the intense feeling of being cold is a remarkably difficult experience for patients. It is observed to occur in 40% to 67% of all postoperative patients [9,18]. Many patients report that the cold sensation and intense shivering are worse than the actual incision and adjacent operative site pain [19]. Vigorous shivering can double or triple oxygen consumption and increase production of carbon dioxide, which further exacerbates normal metabolism and adequate

organ perfusion to kidneys and cardiac muscle [14,18,19].

- Postoperative wound infections cause significant morbidity in postoperative surgical patients. Hypothermia occurring in the perioperative period triggers vasoconstriction, which leads to a decrease in oxygen to traumatized tissues. Tissue oxygen tension is essential for the oxidative destruction of pathogens [18]. To illustrate further the complexities between hypothermia and postoperative wound infections, it is essential to note that shivering caused by hypothermia causes a substantial increase in oxygen consumption to aid the body in heat production at the time that oxygen is most vital to the surgical site [17,18]. Oxygen consumption increases approximately 65% with a decrease in core body temperature of $0.2°C$ $(0.3°F)$ and up to 92% with a reduction in temperature of $0.3°C$ $(0.4°F)$ [17].

A meta-analysis conducted in 1999 concluded that the normothermic surgical patients studied had 64% fewer health care–acquired infections than did the hypothermic cohort [20]. Study results comparing surgical site infections in 200 colorectal procedures showed a 6% infection rate in normothermic patients, whereas patients who experienced mild hypothermia had a 19% infection rate [21]. A host of other studies indicate similar results.

Hypothermia preventive strategies

Multiple studies indicate that maintenance of normothermic conditions throughout the perioperative spectrum results in fewer patient adverse outcomes and decreased health care costs [14]. The American Society of PeriAnesthesia Nurses and the Association of periOperative Registered Nurses have established specific measures to reduce the incidence of perioperative hypothermia. These consistently include

- Identifying patients at risk for hypothermia in the early preoperative phase
- Measuring the patient's temperature throughout the entire perioperative continuum for early detection and early pre-emptive treatment measures
- Specifically observing for shivering, cold extremities, or piloerection
- Using appropriate passive insulation in the form of warm blankets, socks, and head

covering, and minimizing exposure to the surrounding environment

- Early use of active warming strategies including having forced air warming systems, increasing environmental temperature, providing warmed IV fluids and wound irrigation, and humidifying and warming anesthetic gases [14,22–26].

Absent from the literature on hypothermia prevention is the independent variable of the temperature of the resting platforms on which patients are moved during the perioperative course. What is not known is the potential effect on the development of perioperative hypothermia of moving patients on multiple vehicles and whether or not the use of a single device in the pre-, intra-, and postoperative phases would mitigate the onset or the degree to which hypothermia occurs. The overall effect on thermal management of the standard gurney to OR table to PACU bed has not been compared with a single vehicle used for the entire perioperative continuum. The theoretic concept is that most patients will naturally adjust to, and supply body heat to, the surface of the original mattress and coverings in the pre-operative setting at a time when they are the most active and able to generate heat sufficient to create a natural warmth between the transport vehicle surface and the patient. Approximately 30% to 40% of the patient's body surface is in contact with the platform surface. Twenty percent of the thermal input that maintains core temperature is cutaneous [16]. By remaining on the original platform surface through the operative and immediate postoperative phases, one environmental variable of heat loss might be mitigated. The elimination of two cold surfaces at the times that patients are least able to generate heat may reduce the intensity of hypothermia, thermal discomfort, and postoperative shivering.

The recommended practices previously described continue to be valid clinical interventions; however, providing warm cotton blankets has been shown to have little effect on warming patient's core temperatures. The warmth from a heated blanket is lost after 10 minutes and the average number of cotton blankets required has been reported to be nine for each patient [27,28]. Maintaining a patient's thermal comfort is a complex endeavor that requires constant vigilance and nursing assessment. The art and science of the nursing profession is to provide comfort measures for pain and temperature control, to attend to anxiety concerns, and to prevent postoperative complications based on sound supporting evidence. Nursing also seeks to discover new opportunities whenever and wherever possible through evidence-based research methods.

Implications for future research

Further research is needed regarding the effectiveness of single transport-procedure-recovery platforms throughout the continuum of perioperative care with respect to patient safety and comfort and the potential for reducing the incidence of musculoskeletal trauma. No previous studies have considered the implementation of transport-procedure-recovery platforms as a potential influencing variable in the reduction of the occurrence or degree of hypothermia, the economic impact on staff, space requirements, or supply consumption.

Summary

Musculoskeletal injuries among nursing personnel required to lift and laterally transfer patients manually many times daily is well documented and carries substantial injury, salary, and personnel replacement costs per incident. Unintended and unplanned hypothermia in surgical patients has been researched and published with resulting recommendations, yet the problem remains. The primary factor in this phenomenon is the effect of the anesthesia agents used, which universally impact the thermoregulatory mechanisms. Following the appropriate professional recommendations for prevention and treatment of hypothermia is an essential requirement in mitigating the effects of anesthesia and the environmental factors present. Investigating the impact of the multiple cold surfaces of gurneys, OR tables, and recovery platforms on the occurrence of mild hypothermia would seem a logical next step in the discovery of valid solutions.

The primary purpose of this article is to question the potential effects that the use of a single transport-procedure-recovery platform might provide. The full range of surgical care that can be delivered using these platforms has not been explored, in part because of the newness of the concept. Advantages relating to costs, time, space requirements, personnel injury prevention, thermal regulation, nausea and vomiting, biomedical maintenance issues, OR turnover times, fire safety, infection control, and staff and patient satisfaction will not be realized if a specific platform is not able to perform as well as, or better than, the current standard OR tables and allow the performance of most of the procedures currently being performed.

References

[1] Owings MF, Kozak LJ. Ambulatory and inpatient procedures in the United States, 1996. Vital Health Stat 1998;139:1–119.

[2] Nelson A. Safe patient handling and movement: a practical guide for health care professionals. New York: Springer Publishing Company; 2006. p. 67.

[3] Cantrell S. Turning the tables and more: what surgeons and anesthesiologists need in surgical tables. Healthcare Purchasing News April 2007. Available at: http://www.hpnonline.com/inside/2007-04/0704-OR-Tables.html. Accessed September 29, 2007.

[4] Sandburg WS, Canty T, Sokal SM, et al. Financial and operational impact of a direct-from PACU discharge pathway for laparoscopic cholecystectomy patients. Surgery 2006;140(3):372–8.

[5] Sandburg WS, Daily B, Egan M, et al. Deliberate perioperative systems design improves operating room throughput. Anesthesiology 2005;130(2):406–18.

[6] Stahl JE, Sandburg WS, Daily B, et al. Reorganizing patient care and workflow in the operating room: a cost-effectiveness study. Surgery 2006;139(6):717–28.

[7] Krupka DC, Sandburg WS. Operating room design and its impact on operating room economics. Curr Opin Anaesthesiol 2006;19(2):185–91.

[8] Langdon D. Construction cost escalation in California healthcare projects - January 2006. Available at: http://www.calhealth.org/public/press. Accessed October 19, 2007. Accessed September 30, 2007.

[9] Panagiotis K, Poulopoulou M, Argi P, et al. Is postanesthesia care length of stay increased in hypothermic patients? AORN J 2005;81(2):379–92.

[10] AORN. Recommended practices for environmental cleaning in the surgical practice setting. In: Standards, recommended practices, and guidelines. Denver (CO): AORN, Inc.; 2007. p. 551–7.

[11] Bernthal EM. Inadvertent hypothermia prevention: the anaesthetic nurse's role. Br J Nurs 1999;8(1):17–25.

[12] Wagner VD. Unplanned perioperative hypothermia. AORN J 2006;83(2):470–6.

[13] Wagner D, Byrne M, Kolcaba K. Effects of comfort warming on preoperative patients. AORN J 2006;84(3):427–48.

[14] American Society of PeriAnessthesia Nurses. Clinical guideline for the prevention of unplanned perioperative hypothermia. J Perianesth Nurs 2001;16:305–13.

[15] Cooper S. The effects of preoperative warming on patients' postoperative temperatures. AORN J 2006;83(5):1074–84.

[16] Sessler DI. Complications and treatment of mild hypothermia. Anesthesiology 2001;95:531–43.

[17] Good KK, Verble JA, Norwood BR. Postoperative hypothermia—the chilling consequences. AORN J 2006;83(5):1055–66.

[18] Sessler DI. Perioperative thermoregulation and heat balance. Ann N Y Acad Sci 1997;813(1):757–74.

[19] DeWitte J, Sessler DI. Perioperative shivering; physiology and pharmacology. Anesthesiology 2002;96:467–84.

[20] Mahoney J, Odom J. Maintaining intraoperative normotherma: a meta-analysis of outcomes with costs. J Am Assoc Nurse Anesth 1999;67:155–63.

[21] Braxton C. The surgical infection prevention and surgical care improvement projects. 12th Annual Kansas Health Quality Forum: March 2007. Available at: http://www.kfmc.org/providers/CPE/completed/QF2007/presentations/Dr.%20Braxton_QF.pdf. Accessed October 19, 2007.

[22] AORN. Recommended practices for safe care through identification of potential hazards in the surgical environment. In: Standards, recommended practices, and guidelines. Denver (CO): AORN, Inc.; 2007. p. 575–81.

[23] Blanchard J, Mitchell S. Clinical issues: preventing unplanned perioperative hypothermia. AORN J 2007;86(4):660–1.

[24] Brendle TA. Surgical care improvement project and the perioperative nurse's role. AORN J 2007;86(1):94–101.

[25] Bitner J, Hilde L, Hall K, et al. A team approach to the prevention of unplanned postoperative hypothermia. AORN J 2007;85(5):921–9.

[26] Recommended practices for the prevention of unplanned perioperative hypothermia. AORN J 2007;85(5):972–88.

[27] Sessler DI, Schroeder M. Heat loss in humans covered with cotton hospital blankets. Anesth Analg 1993;77:73–7.

[28] Senn GF. Some cold, hard facts about warmed cotton blankets. SSM 2002;8:19–25.

ELSEVIER
SAUNDERS

Perioperative Nursing Clinics 3 (2008) 43–54

PERIOPERATIVE
NURSING
CLINICS

Planning a Better Operating Room Suite: Design and Implementation Strategies for Success

Randy Tomaszewski, RN, BSN, MBA

Skytron, 5085 Corporate Exchange Boulevard SE, Grand Rapids, MI 49512, USA

Whether your operating room (OR) design project involves renovation, new construction, or a little of both, OR equipment layout planning and implementation strategies can be challenging, with available technologies representing a staggering array of options. Although many equipment choices, floor plans, and solutions are available, having a clear understanding of your own facility's future goals is a big step toward arriving at the best solution to meet your facility's growth needs.

Assembling a qualified, multidisciplinary hospital team in guiding decisions pays big dividends later on, when clinical staff and other team members actually begin using or supporting activities in the OR suite. Trusted representatives from your key support staff are essential to your decision-making team. Examples include, but are not limited to, surgeons; nurse managers; hospital administrators; purchasing, anesthesia, and nursing team leaders; scrub and circulating nurses; perfusionists; surgical technicians; information technology and biomedical engineers; an equipment planner; and your selected architect, who will be creating the design plan and infrastructure to support your overall plan. A well-coordinated team approach to planning your OR suite will deliver the highest probability for success and acceptance, including implementation once the planning is done. Proper timing and excellent clinical planning translate into OR construction and renovation projects that come in on time, on target, and within budget.

Planning and successful system implementation requires an interdisciplinary team that works closely with suppliers from the very beginning. Bring together various stakeholders so that all interests are considered (eg, nursing, OR, purchasing, IT and biomedical engineering). You should include vendors in particular whom you are considering to provide your surgical facility booms and lights and providers for your endoscopic products [1].

A well-designed, functional, and flexible project requires 2 to 3 years of well-coordinated team planning for the best results. Start from your goal date and work backward to identify critical milestones that must be met to hit your target opening date. To be safe, a good rule of thumb is to plan on a 6-month lead time for selected vendors to deliver equipment you have specified to build, ship, and install, which means that decisions about room design and sign-offs of critical engineering drawings must be in place no later than 6 months before your opening date. Construction and preparation for mounting structures and support infrastructure should be made before that. Otherwise, as the old saying goes, changing an architectural drawing on paper in the early planning stages may cost you a few hundred dollars, but midway through the planning process the same change may cost thousands of dollars. Last-minute changes can cost your facility tens to hundreds of thousands of dollars; such costs could have been avoided with better communication, time allocation, and team planning and coordination.

Care should be taken in your overall OR design plan to build on the advantages that booms and flat-panel display arms deliver for efficient and optimally flexible OR integration solutions (now or in the future). OR integration technologies can convert the complex world of

E-mail address: rtomaszewski@skytron.us

video and data routing, communication, and control into one simple-to-use, instant-access control tool with instant-response, video-confirmation capability, before critical video images and clinical data are routed and displayed for the surgeon and surgical team (Fig. 1). Multiple display monitors surrounding the surgical field ensure that surgeons have the optimal and comfortable viewing line of site for highest-quality high-definition interoperative digital video (minimally invasive surgery [MIS], picture archiving and communication systems [PACS], C-arm, computerized information), including speedy on-board instant image capture capability and streaming video. Bidirectional teleconferencing and more are also easily made available. Your integration control system should provide the same level of flexibility and open architecture design and multi-source video and data management including MIS images, in-room and surgical light cameras, PACS, C-arm, microscopes, HIS, Internet, radiology, electronic medical records (EMR), teleconferencing, 3-D stereotactics, digital imaging and more.

Hospitals should realize in the early stages of planning that integration is quickly becoming a requirement, not optional. Space must be allotted for equipment that will be needed, plans for wiring and conduit for each source and destination location. Time added to design planning for each task required must be included at specific stages of construction. Failure to plan and budget accordingly will almost definitely result in delays [1].

Operating rooms are quickly becoming an informational hub. Integrated ORs are a fast growing trend. Welcome to the world of EMR, PACS and the integrated MP3 player. Although referred to as digital ORs, it is more appropriate to refer to them as integrated or automated operating rooms because most of the routed signals are analog video and it is simply the control of the system components that is digital (the term digital is thrown around because it is a popular buzz word). The integrated OR is not a product. What you are purchasing from the vendor is the brain (hub, user interfaces, etc.) that tie together all of the other companies' products. Integrating multiple devices results in changes of workflow and requires creation of a nursing command center within each OR. From this seat, the nurse can control images and other data to various monitors around the OR. The nurse cannot only access and update patient information, but can route this information for others in real time. In simplest terms, the integrated OR is intended to route signals from

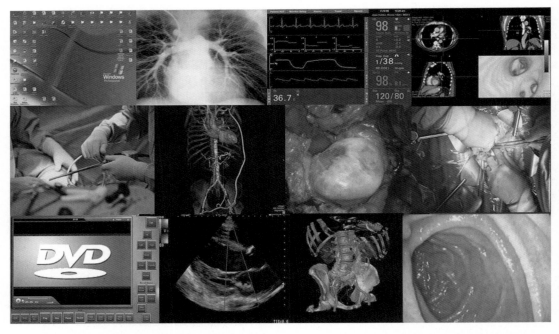

Fig. 1. OR integration and the delivery of advanced communications, picture archiving and communication systems, multivideo displays, data, and electronic medical records to the surgical field. (*Courtesy of* Skytron, Grand Rapids, MI.)

one location (the source) to another (the destination). The most common source for images is endoscopic video cameras, radiographic images (via the PACS), patient vital signs or even the internet browser. This information can be displayed on any destination attached to the system, whether a boom-mounted display or large-screen, wall-mounted plasma display. The information can also be routed locally in one OR to between multiple ORs, conference rooms and other remote locations – creating ways to teach and consult not available just a few years ago [1].

Each facility must decide for itself the advantages of video integration solutions. One must determine the hospital's long-term information technology goal and budget. Some systems are compatible with multiple vendors, providing open architecture solutions, whereas others are not. An evaluation of the right integration system for your facility should consider cost, ease of use, whether the architecture is open, and future adaptability, and should be in line with the mission statement of your facility. Obtaining the greatest value and greatest overall flexibility for present and future growth is key, including adaptable, flexible, and user-friendly designs delivering state-of-the-art services for your surgical team.

Clearly define your clinical goals and specify the level of integration desired. Most integrated OR suppliers meet the typical requirements for a facility's expected surgical workflow, storage, remote image distribution, security and management functions. However, there are notable differences in the manner in which these suppliers meet specific requirements of individual facilities and differences related to reliability and support [1].

Ease of use and ease of installation should be considered in the final selection of the integration system. One should ask how many hard drives are required in each room to install and support the system and its platform and how much cabling is required to be run to each source and destination. Some integration systems are simple and efficient, and require far less cabling and conduit to establish source-to-destination communication; they also manage signals from the communications hub and display the signals to 1280 × 1024, the native resolution for flat-panel displays, before pushing the data from source to destination monitors. The signal arriving at the monitor in this case is already at its native resolution and has been automatically "prescreened" beforehand by the nurse circulator before routing to the surgeon, providing an immediately crisp, clear, and

representative image to native image at the surgical field. The native image (the image produced at the source [ie, MIS camera, C-arm, surgical light camera, and so forth]) typically is routed to multiple video designations elsewhere within the OR. Video display monitors typically display reference images from the original primary source by optimizing the video display to its native resolution of 1280 × 1024, which typically is the most efficient video resolution for each flat panel display to provide a crisp, clear reference image from the original. These systems also require far fewer cables to route, install, and maintain, eliminating the need to run multiple cables through conduit and booms, which unnecessarily packs the internal diameter with communications cables in addition to those for other key services such as medical gas and electric, a situation that can lead to cable damage and signal loss and that can make the boom more difficult to move.

Each cable pulled is billed for, including the cable itself and its installation, and the installation process itself is also lengthened. Routing data, video, PACS, and other signals directly to the flat-panel display, versus converting to the 1280 × 1024 native resolution of the flat-panel display, can also create a potential lag, in that the monitor itself has to convert signals internally before the correct format is obtained. This process can lead to a temporary delay of the data, video, or PACS image at the flat-panel display supporting the surgeon and surgical team, which can lead to surgeon and staff frustration, especially if the image is displayed incorrectly.

Surgical lighting advances with light-emitting diode technology

The latest advancement in surgical lighting is light-emitting diode (LED) surgical lighting technology. Surgeons and the entire surgical team can now benefit from the bright, high-quality lighting intensity produced by LED surgical lights with minimal heat output compared with competitive, traditional halogen systems. LED lighting technology requires significantly less energy to power the lighting system (an energy-saving technology) and LEDs last a minimum of 10 years (ie, no more bulbs burning out or having to be changed during surgery). LED lighting systems are also cool to work under, even for extended cases (such as cardiovascular surgery and neurosurgery), owing to low heat and power requirements. Some LED surgical lighting systems also permit the surgeon to select preferred temperatures for each case; the lighting systems can also be camera equipped (Fig. 2).

Basic operating room design

OR design plans, with the exception of those for some specialties such as cardiovascular, orthopedics, and urology, are designed for maximum flexibility, to accommodate as many different types of surgical cases as possible. Each OR should be evaluated with design goals to enhance and accelerate start times, throughput, and overall efficiency. "The creation of an optimally functional space starts before actual design and construction of the facility begins," according to John F. Stephan, AIA, senior project architect with Marshall Erdman & Associates. "Advanced planning is really the key to making everything work well; getting together with the people who are going to use the space to talk about what their plans are, near term and long term. If we know exactly what it is they are going to be doing, procedure-wise, that helps us with the flexibility of the space as well" [2].

With the advancement of MIS techniques now covering every surgical discipline, today's ORs have become highly advanced technologic wonders by standards measured 20 years ago. However, the equipment demands and location requirements to support multiple surgical disciplines in this advanced, flexible, technologic, and user-friendly environment require well-thought-out planning that considers the needs for each procedure.

Space and square footage come at a premium in today's OR designs. Most newly constructed ORs require a minimum of 600 square feet or larger, with a recommended finished ceiling height of 10 feet. This size and height are ideal to deliver advanced equipment and integration technologies for the twenty-first century and beyond.

> At one time, a 400 sq. ft. operating room seemed huge. Now with all the technology found in ORs, there's barely room for the patient. Six hundred sq. ft. rooms are being planned for future technology and growth. It is much easier to train in larger rooms and staff is able to focus more on patient care [3].

Just as important as ceiling height and square footage to today's modern ORs is the available space between the finished and structural ceiling, commonly known as the plenum space. The distance between the two should be at least 3 feet, with an absolute minimum no less than 18 in, because utility services (medical gases, electric circuits, and communications cabling and conduits) are running in this space. Ideally, access to these areas should be made available, even after the ceiling is closed, by way of an access panel, or from above the finished ceiling by way of a catwalk or crawl space, so as to be in the best position to adapt to future technologies and OR design changes. "Make sure your OR has enough conduits, electrical power and ceiling structure to support new and emerging technology. Running extra pipe and conduits into ORs during construction can also help you prepare for the future," says architect Thomas Harvey of HKS, Inc. in Dallas. Higher ceilings can also be an important factor to consider in planning for the future. With more equipment being suspended from the ceiling, a ceiling height of 10 feet to 10 and a half feet may be more suitable, say experts [4].

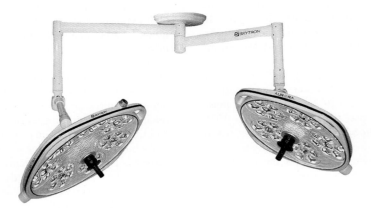

Fig. 2. Aurora LED surgical lighting system. (*Courtesy of* Skytron, Grand Rapids, MI.)

Mounting structures: location, location, location

Providing optimal flexibility

General and orthopedic ORs have traditionally had surgical lights directly over the surgical table. In contrast, medical gas and electric services were delivered at the head and foot of the surgical table for anesthesia and nurse circulators, with video carts positioned to the left and right sides of the surgical table, depending on the procedure being performed. For specialty procedures such as cardiovascular surgery, more surgical staff and equipment were required, including target support for the perfusionists, surgical assistants, anesthetist, surgeons, and scrub and circulating nurses.

Mounted in the right locations, surgical lighting, booms, and flat-panel display arms can greatly enhance OR design flexibility and support of the entire surgical team. The benefit is the elimination of the footprint and floor clutter created by MIS equipment towers, cables, cords, and hoses or the need for secondary monitor carts for assisting surgeons. Mounting these devices safely on equipment carriers and within enclosed arm sets (that can rotate to specific target areas with little effort to position) also significantly reduces damage to equipment and potential injury to surgical staff, who would otherwise have to push, pull, or lift, or may trip over items to get them in the right position. Turnover and set-up times are also significantly reduced when floor clutter is reduced or eliminated.

Ask any real estate agent what the top three real estate priorities are and they will quickly tell you "location, location, location." Located in the right place, real estate value is maximized. In no greater arena does this fundamental play a more significant role than within the OR. The flexibility of the OR design, its efficiency, speed of set up, usage, and overall construction costs all are directly related to proper mounting locations, user-friendliness, and the overall simplicity versus complexity of the OR design (Fig. 3).

When purchasing booms, consider the future adaptability of the product. Two questions you might ask the supplier: How will the piece of equipment adapt to future technologies? How is the company thinking of the future in design of their equipment? By understanding how the company is preparing for the future, you can determine whether or not the long-term investment will hold up several years down the road [4].

Optimal OR design is not one in which one takes all the clutter that was on the floor and creates as much, or more, clutter by placing several mounting structures on the ceiling. Usually, the more mounting structures, the less flexibility to accommodate multiple procedures. Fewer, well-placed mounting structures create greater overall flexibility in non-dedicated (and dedicated) room designs.

Today's efficient OR designs must be flexible for every case, not just for some. Otherwise, start times are negatively impacted, patients must be rotated to use the equipment properly, and surgical staff

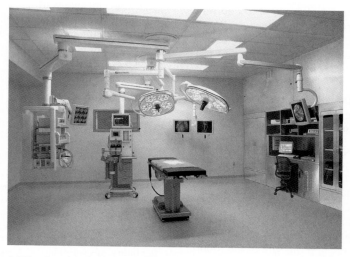

Fig. 3. Fully integrated OR suite with lights, boom, and multiple flat-panel displays capable of displaying multivideo images, PACS, fluoroscopy, electronic medical records, and more, with a dedicated nurse documentation center for OR integration control. (*Courtesy of* Skytron, Grand Rapids, MI.)

must reposition to support the patient and surgical team properly; safety and infection can be concerns with frequent patient position changes; and the efficiency of the OR itself (and the ease of suspended equipment use) can be reduced by using poorly positioned mounting structures.

Special considerations regarding booms for anesthesia

The dedicated needs of anesthesia should always be considered separately from those of the surgeon and other boom users, including the positioning requirements to support equipment and monitors in multiple locations. Anesthesia requires dedicated services (medical gas, communications, power outlets, data, and phone) delivered to a key target separate from other booms. The only exception would be to consider adding a separate flat-panel display arm to an anesthesia boom-mounting structure (either for anesthesia's use or as a secondary video image for the surgeon), equipped with a single or side-by-side video display, available for use around the surgical field at the head end of the surgical table. In short, anesthesia needs its own boom in every OR design.

Today's OR designs and enhanced flexibility should eliminate, or at least keep to a minimum, the requirement of 180° patient rotation. Any time a patient has to be rotated or repositioned, a domino effect occurs that impacts the entire surgical team. Anesthesia has to reposition, access to supplies for the circulating nurse and her/his pathway to and from have to be rethought, sterile field considerations must be reviewed with regard to doorways and traffic points in the OR, start times are delayed because set up for the procedure takes longer, surgical turns are slowed from procedure to procedure, and the efficiency of the OR is decreased.

History lessons of the 1980s and 1990s: laterally positioned mounting structures for booms (three and nine o'clock positioning)

Early boom designs, and the mounting structures to support them, followed user positioning locations for carts, utilities, and service target areas, including mounts off the head of the surgical table for anesthesia, off the foot of the table for the circulating nurse (or, if the patient was rotated 180°, for anesthesia, with the circulating nurse using the boom at the opposite end of the room). Typically, dual surgical lights were mounted directly over the surgical table. With the onset of MIS and endoscopic equipment on carts, the desire

was to position boom-mounting structures in the same locations, with a high value placed on storing equipment up against the wall when not needed. Chief among the limited MIS surgical cases being performed 20 years ago was the lap chole MIS procedure; this procedure required an equipment boom over the patient's left shoulder to support large, heavy cathode ray tube monitors and equipment, including cameras, light sources, insufflators, videocassette recorders, and printers, and another boom over the patient's right shoulder to hold a separate monitor for the assisting surgeon (Fig. 4).

Location problems with boom mounts used in the late 1980s and 1990s were multiple: (1) simply moving the clutter from the floor to the ceiling accomplished little; (2) equipment used a decade ago was much larger and heavier, requiring a large boom to replace video carts, which was hard to move and hard to store, (3) MIS equipment, monitors, and services were limited to one side of the operating room or surgical field. Redundancy and duplication of services to provide availability to both sides of the room based upon original design limitations required added expenses for multiple mounting structures, more installation time and labor, and for more ceiling clutter. Multiple mounting structures in the ceiling, in turn, created potential obstructions and efficiency problems in moving patients, carts, and portable C-arms in and out of ORs and created the need to navigate through a suspended maze of equipment. Earlier boom room designs blocked doorways and supply cabinets. The goal of storing an equipment carrier on a wall or in a low-traffic area when not in use was costly and inflexible. Moving and positioning large heavy booms loaded with equipment made use of the booms difficult.

> Today's booms are more flexible, lighter weight and smaller in size, making them sleek and easy to move for any and every procedure. Booms mounted centrally with equipment carriers, flat panels and lights provide an even greater flexibility advantage case to case. These systems provide optimal flexibility and efficiencies in delivering illumination, video images, equipment and services exactly where surgeons and the surgical team need them [5].

Operating room design improvements: the flexibility of evolution and keeping it simple

Today, boom designs have become much smaller owing to the advancements in the design

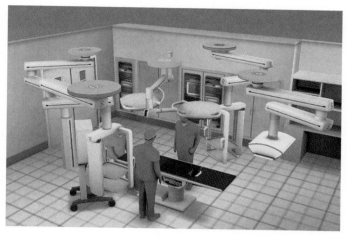

Fig. 4. Cluttered ceiling with early boom designs of the 1980s and 1990s at head and foot for support of anesthesia and circulating nurse, with surgical lights mounted over the surgical table. Equipment carrier booms mounted laterally (at three and nine o'clock positions). (*Courtesy of* Skytron, Grand Rapids, MI.)

of the equipment to be housed on them. Much improved and flexible OR designs are possible today, requiring fewer booms and the separate delivery of flat-panel display arms for video, PACS, and fluoroscopy images, which can be quickly moved into position and up overhead when not required, allowing less clutter, fewer mounting structures, and optimal positioning flexibility for every procedure.

> The technology revolution continues in minimally invasive surgery. As MIS techniques continue to evolve, systems and instruments are designed smaller and more compact. They take up less space in the OR and combine technology to further cost effectiveness [6].

The history of surgical light positioning has consistently indicated that lighting should be mounted over the surgical table to deliver surgical lighting needs efficiently in a circumferential delivery area from a central point of positioning for maximum flexibility for any procedure. Owing to advancements in boom designs and reductions in the size and weight of support equipment, ceiling-mounted booms can now also be centrally mounted with surgical lights and flat-panel displays, optimizing the same positioning efficiencies surgical lighting has always provided over the center of the surgical table (Fig. 5).

With the flexibility available in today's boom designs, equipment can be positioned to reach key target areas, with fewer, optimally positioned mounting structures.

The size and weight of medical equipment have been reduced significantly. Printers today can be wired and cabled outside the surgical field. Cameras, insufflators, light sources, shavers, and so forth, are much smaller and lighter than ever before. One of the most defining changes making OR suites more flexible is the evolution and quality of flat-panel displays versus large and heavy cathode ray tube monitors. Flat-panel displays allow for far greater positioning options for images in and around the surgical field, including PACS, high-definition video, fluoroscopy images, and more. Because nurses typically are required to move and position booms and monitors, compact, lightweight booms and flat-panel displays are most favorable for individuals of smaller stature and strength, preventing back strain and injuries from lifting or pushing.

Low ceiling height or air handling system accommodations

Split-mount (twelve and six o'clock) mounting structure positioning

Booms and flat-panel displays today are capable of being mounted on fewer structures (together with surgical lights), providing greater options for optimal flexibility. Split mounts have often been used for specialty surgical disciplines such as cardiovascular and orthopedic surgery, where more than two surgical lights may be used. Similar strategies can be used to optimize positioning

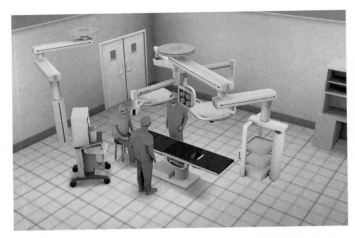

Fig. 5. OR suite design with optimally flexible ceiling-mounted equipment (surgical lights, boom, flat-panel displays) capable of positioning at any point around the entire periphery of the surgical table and patient. (*Courtesy of* Skytron, Grand Rapids, MI).

flexibility for low ceiling height (less than 10 ft) or for working with airflow circulation grids positioned over the surgical field, which still provide optimal coverage owing to the enhanced reach of new surgical light radial arms, flat-panel display, and boom arms. Splitting mounting structures to head and foot locations still maintains optimal flexibility to deliver surgical lighting, video images, equipment, and services to either side of the surgical field, even with lower ceiling heights (Fig. 6).

A second option for the delivery of lighting, flat-panel displays, and booms is the lateral three and nine o'clock positioning. Anesthesia is dedicated and is mounted separately off the head end of the surgical table. However, drawbacks of this option are that an additional mounting structure is required and the equipment carrier range is limited to one side and the foot end of the surgical table. Additionally, patients and equipment brought into and out of the surgical room are potentially

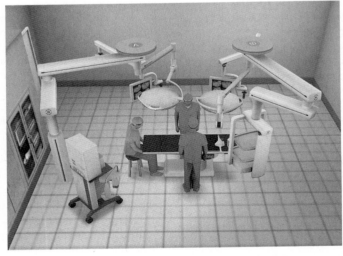

Fig. 6. Low ceiling height OR suite design, featuring flexible ceiling-mounted equipment on split mounting structures over head and foot of the surgical table. Surgical lights, boom, and flat-panel displays are capable of bilateral positioning around the entire periphery of the surgical table and patient. (*Courtesy of* Skytron, Grand Rapids, MI.)

obstructed by the equipment carrier requiring frequent movement, as illustrated in Fig. 7.

Wireless radio frequency identification real-time awareness tracking systems

Yet another advance in OR suite design is the deployment of wireless radio frequency identification (RFID) for tracking staff and equipment can be made within the OR suite (Fig. 8). Tracking processes and improving efficiencies and improvements in processes can be made by studying patient flows; studying the reduction in search time for surgical table accessories such as orthopedic spine devices and specialty surgical instrument sets; real-time awareness of OR openings; and more. Wireless RFID is the latest technologic advancement showing great promise in improving surgical equipment and staff processes and efficiencies. Wireless RFID tracking systems provide real-time location, status, and movement of equipment, people, and information, with maximum impact and minimum disruption; are designed to map, monitor, measure, and improve processes and efficiencies of equipment and people; and improve the performance and use of critical resources, thereby lessening time requirements and improving safety, patient care, and overall profitability.

New construction or renovation: mounting structure testing

Adequately built mounting structures are the key to any fixed equipment's ability to provide years of reliable positioning, case after case. It is essential that the architect have the mounting structure requirements and moment loads of the boom and lighting systems you intend to deploy in your new facility. Suspended equipment systems change position dynamically from case to case, based on the positioning requirements of the surgeon and surgical team. Therefore, the mounting structures cannot have any slop or flex, or the equipment will "drift." In either case (new construction versus renovation), once the ceiling is closed by the architect or contractor and the room opens, it is far too late to address mounting structure limitations, without heavy costs. Building and testing mounting structures to a dynamic maximum load is the best way to ensure optimal equipment performance.

Hospital and vendor site visits

Visiting other hospital facilities that have also planned and designed ORs to meet the ever-increasing demands of today's most demanding surgical procedures is highly recommended. The opportunity to learn from testimonials about the hard lessons learned by others and about the excellent benefits that the facility is reaping from good design practice is well worth your decision-making team's time. Map, monitor, measure, improve is a good practice to use when going on site visits. Finding out what the facility did right or wrong can help tremendously in arriving at your own successful OR suite design. However, each facility also has its own set of physical,

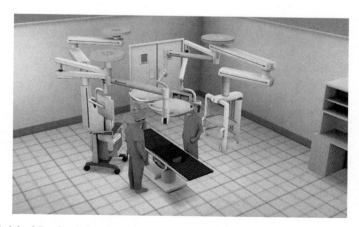

Fig. 7. Low ceiling height OR suite design, featuring ceiling-mounted equipment on split mounting structures on lateral sides (three and nine o'clock) of the surgical table. This design requires an additional mounting structure and has less overall flexibility. (*Courtesy of* Skytron, Grand Rapids, MI.)

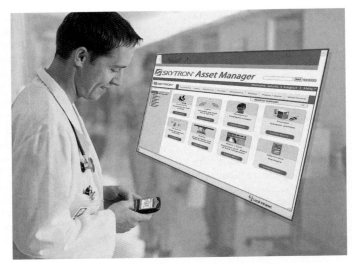

Fig. 8. Wireless RFID for support of RFID asset tracking technology. (*Courtesy of* Skytron, Grand Rapids, MI.)

budgetary, and clinical objectives based on its particular needs. Look for symmetry and overlap in shared goals versus limitations or even over-indulgences in design you don't feel your facility needs. Other potential drawbacks include the time you'll actually be allowed to review the equipment and visit with clinicians, which will depend on their patient load on a particular day, or how dated a project is, compared to better technology that is now available.

> Figure out what you're going to use the ORs for now and a few years down the road. Will they be used strictly for surgery or will teaching also take place? What types of data will be sent and received? What kinds of surgery will be performed? By knowing how the ORs will be used, you can better plan for what types of equipment you may need in the future [4].

Visiting vendor sites and showrooms provides another perspective, which is beneficial to the decision-making team. Here, more time is available to work with the equipment physically and to ask questions. Typically, showrooms are set up with a better and best approach that shows not only today's designs but trends and product improvement ideas based on customer clinical feedback for future designs of tomorrow. Although the clinical feedback of users is not typically available at a vendor site visit, the product management team has most likely talked with several hospitals and is aware of trends and

solutions best suited to meet evolving clinical needs. The product presentational team is typically the best informed about the product, with its equipment and overall menu of solutions designed around your identified clinical needs.

Three-dimensional floor plans from prospective vendors or architect

Most medical equipment suppliers and architects have the ability to represent their product in three dimensions to allow the decision-making team to see what each product solution could look like to scale in its own OR, complete with walls, cabinetry, doorways, patient entry, back tables, and so forth. The vendor or architect can provide this powerful design tool as a service in planning the most flexible and suitable OR design to best meet your overall team's clinical and business objectives. In addition, this tool can be taken on site at your facility for input not only from team participants but also from surgeons and other key surgical team members unable to make a visit, with good discussion and feedback based on favored designs and discovery (Fig. 9).

> 3D software can save months of planning and help you equip the room of your dreams. Software that lets you drag and drop equipment into an animated suite that is the exact size and shape of the one you're building promises to greatly improve the efficiency of the OR design process [7].

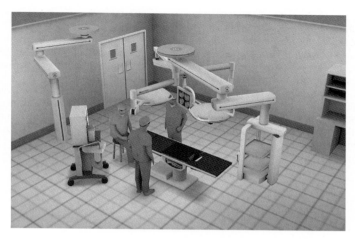

Fig. 9. Three-dimensional OR design tool. (*Courtesy of* Skytron, Grand Rapids, MI.)

Mock operating rooms

Booms, in particular, are next to impossible to "demo" because plumbing in medical gas lines for gas outlets, electric and video routing, and certification, and mounting the appropriate structure are cost prohibitive and impractical to do "live," beyond mounting a set of surgical lights and a flat-panel monitor or monitors. However, some facilities decide that the best way to know for sure, if they have the budget available, is to designate a mock OR and walk people through for design and clinical feedback. Here again is a tool designed to validate and provide for participants who will eventually be impacted every day by OR design decisions that they might not otherwise have had the opportunity to review, touch, and feel. This mock OR can be set up by building mounting structures for real equipment (and not running gas hoses, and so forth) off site but within reasonable distance of the hospital facility, using plastic piping or other model materials for distances, and mounting in locations according to clinical team needs, or by having the vendor bring in mounting truss legs and apparatus to hang the equipment properly at an off- or on-site facility for review. The benefit here is no mounting structure costs and that a reasonable positioning of the equipment floor plan can be temporarily supported by a truss grid designed to hold the weight of the ceiling-mounted equipment. Mock ORs can be expensive to pursue, but, in the minds of some hospital decision makers, the investment to be right far outweighs the potential to buy unseen and be wrong.

The final goal

The measure of success in planning for new construction or renovation projects lies in the success of implementation after the design phase is over. If the project is well planned and the right feedback is achieved, it should meet specified goals for growth and provide for future growth needs with a plan that looks forward at least 10 years. The most successful plan involves a team effort and multidisciplinary input from key clinical end users and support personnel. The goal should always be maximum flexibility and adaptability to anticipated future needs, and the ability to perform as many surgical procedures as possible within the same OR with ease, enhanced throughput, and accelerated start times. The OR should also have a standardized environment that is familiar for your surgical staff and that considers all surgical disciplines that will be involved, including future surgical specialties planned. Technologically advanced OR solutions should enhance and optimize surgical practice, flexibility, efficiency, and safety within multifunctional, state-of-the-art surgical suites you can be proud of for years to come, and your project should be delivered on time and within budget.

References

[1] Renton D. Minimally invasive surgery. Compact designs and improved instrumentation continue the MIS revolution. Outpatient Surgery Magazine. July 2007 Guide to New Products for Surgery. p. 26.

[2] Strong J. Emerging technology. The Source, Official Magazine of Healthtrust 2007;2(1):6–9, 32, 33.

[3] Miller M. Equipping your OR for the future. As minimally invasively surgery evolves, the integrated surgical suite will become the new standard of care. Outpatient Surgery Magazine. 2007 Mnager's Guide to New Surgical Construction. p. 54–64.

[4] Taylor D. If I could redo my OR. Outpatient Surgery Magazine. June 2006. p. 32–40.

[5] Ellis K, Planning the perfect space. The effort to build in clinical efficiency and flexibility. Available at: http://www.surgicenteronline.com. Accessed August 11, 2007.

[6] Ross K, Pinkney N. The rise of the automated operating room pulling IT all together in the OR. Medical Construction & Design Journal. January/February 2007. p. 16–9.

[7] Hockersmith L. What will your ORs look like in 2017? How to plan in the present for the operating suite of the future. Outpatient Surgery Magazine. January 2007 Manager's Guide to New Surgical Reconstruction. p. 80–6.

ELSEVIER
SAUNDERS

Perioperative Nursing Clinics 3 (2008) 55–62

PERIOPERATIVE
NURSING
CLINICS

Perioperative Facility Planning Considerations

Susan M. Myers, RN, MSN*, Kevin Schlaht, AIA, MArch, MBA

The Innova Group, 800 South Austin Avenue, Suite M, Georgetown, TX 78626, USA

In 2006, the cost per square foot for hospital construction averaged between $265 and $275 nationwide [1]. In January of 2006 in California, hospital construction costs per square foot were as high as $550 [2]. "The hospital industry has spent nearly $100 billion in inflation-adjusted dollars in the past five years on new facilities, up 47% from the previous five years, according to the Census Bureau" [3]. Because of the significant financial investment in health care facility construction, it is critical to ensure that each resulting facility meets the needs of users and is flexible in design to allow for changes that occur in health care delivery systems over time. The process for health care facility planning is lengthy, ranging from 2 to 7 years, and includes the following critical steps: initial identification that a facility is needed; definition of how health care will be delivered in the new facility by all users; development of a design that supports the planned functions, construction of the facility; and occupancy by the users. Too often, clinical input into the design of the facility is inadequate in ensuring that the end product is a functional space for the patients and supports intended processes. Also, if clinical input is provided too late in the facility development continuum, changes to facility design can become either costly or not feasible. Clinical input into health care facility design must be included from the inception of the new facility idea to ensure a functionally supportive and usable facility in the end.

Perioperative services is an inherently high-cost department in new facility construction. Effectively planning this department early in the facility-development process can minimize avoidable and expensive late stage facility construction costs. A global view of facility health care operations is required to plan adequately for perioperative support areas because users come from throughout the health care facility. This global view would require knowledge of the organization's impact on specific perioperative support areas, each of which is discussed in detail: preadmissions, preoperative processing, operating room (OR) support areas, equipment and supply storage for surgical suites, and postanesthesia care unit (PACU) requirements for phase I and phase II recovery. Differences in planning for these perioperative support areas in a large hospital venue, versus an ambulatory surgery center venue, are also highlighted.

Preadmissions

Preadmissions functions vary from one organization to another and have evolved as the percentage of ambulatory procedures has come to dominate the total number of procedures performed in a facility. Generally, the role of preadmissions is to compile nursing assessments, physician's health histories, surgical procedure consent forms, laboratory results, radiographs, EKGs, and any other documentation that has to be completed and available before the start of any surgical procedure or invasive intervention.

For some preadmissions units, the function is merely an administrative exercise requiring office space to interview patients and compile surgical charts and to provide patient waiting space. Other preadmissions units serve as a "one-stop-shop," drawing preoperative blood work, performing EKGs, and conducting anesthesia assessments before the day of the procedure. In organizations

* Corresponding author. 1714 Cactus Bluff, San Antonio, TX 78258.

E-mail address: susan.myers@theinnovagroup.com (S.M. Myers).

where orthopedic procedures are performed, incorporating an area to teach crutch walking to those patient requiring crutches postoperatively should also be considered. When planning this area, one may also want to take into consideration the provision of consultation spaces for other health care team members to consult with patients. For instance, patients undergoing mastectomy, gastric bypass, or other complicated and life-changing procedures may benefit from having the opportunity to speak with psychologists, nutritionists, social workers, and so forth, during the preadmissions process. All these functions require spaces designed specifically for the activities to be performed, while still allowing for patient privacy. Planning for preadmissions functions, whether in an ambulatory surgery center or a hospital setting, necessitates a clear understanding of the scope of services to be provided. The clinical services that will use the preadmissions process ultimately drives the number of patients who will be processed daily. This critical calculation enables planning for a sufficient number of appropriately designed and sized support spaces.

Preoperative processing

Preoperative processing functions use spaces needed from the time a patient arrives on the day of a scheduled procedure until the time he/she is transferred to the surgical suite or area where the intervention will occur. Activities incorporated in this process include reception, patient and family waiting, family counseling, preoperative preparation, and, possibly, premedication for procedures. Once again, understanding which clinical activities will send patients through this area, quantifying the volume of patients flowing through this area daily, and defining processes that patients and staff will perform during this time, defines the number and types of spaces needed [4]. This information applies to ambulatory surgery centers and hospital-based services.

Reception is the first function the patient interfaces with on the day of a procedure. This area requires adequate space to accommodate the receptionists and storage for any files, charts, or forms necessary to service patients as they arrive. Additionally, the reception area must afford some level of auditory privacy as patients communicate with receptionists concerning the purpose of their visit.

A waiting area designed for patients' family members and significant others will likely be in the same immediate area as reception. Generally, this area also serves as a patient waiting area until the patient is taken to a more private preoperative preparation area. In the meantime, the patient's family and significant others will remain in the waiting room during the patient's procedure and recovery process and until the patient is ready to go home. Understanding the daily volume of patient procedures and the average number of family members patients bring with them is critical to making this environment functional and comfortable. The demographics of the primary service area population, coupled with an analysis of health care system users, will indicate whether patients are more likely to bring one person with them or multiple family members.

The waiting area should also have private rooms for consultation with the physician and family immediately after the procedure. Generally, the physician will come to the waiting area to update the family or significant other regarding how the procedure went and the condition of the patient. Patient and family privacy is a great concern and such communications should be conducted in private, separately from the open waiting area. The number of private consultation rooms needed depends on the volume of procedures being conducted daily.

Staff directs the patient from the waiting area to the preoperative preparation area. This area provides privacy for the patient to change into hospital attire and be interviewed by nursing and anesthesia staff in preparation for his/her procedure. The processes used by the staff to care for the patient will impact how this area is designed.

One option provides men's and women's locker rooms for changing into and out of hospital attire and secured locker spaces for storage of personal clothing items. Patients then proceed to a private "bed" area where they can wait comfortably on a gurney or reclining chair. This area is where the preoperative interviews are conducted. This locker room concept allows the preoperative areas to be used by multiple patients because each "bed" is vacated when patients move to their procedure rooms. These areas should have private toilet facilities for patient use, either in the rooms themselves or immediately adjacent.

Another option ushers the patient into a private "bed" area where he/she can change into hospital attire. This area can still be used by multiple patients, simply by having their belongings bagged and labeled to stay with each patient through the perioperative process. This process omits the need for locker rooms, while still allowing bed spaces to be used by multiple patients. Ideally, these areas would have private toilet facilities in each room.

A third option assigns a private "bed" area to one patient throughout his/her stay during the perioperative process. The private "bed" area has clothes storage and the patient returns to this same room for phase II recovery. Ideally, these areas should have private toilet facilities in each room. This option is seldom used, however, because of the sizeable space requirement and the fact that each "bed" area goes unused for significant time periods during the day.

Part of the preoperative process involves starting the intravenous line, administrating preoperative medications, and placing regional blocks. Preoperative medications can include sedative medications and antibiotics. When sedative medications are administered, the staff's ability to monitor the patient and respond should the patient become oversedated is a significant safety concern. Patients undergoing placement of regional blocks in the preoperative processing area will also require close monitoring and immediate access by staff after block placement to respond to alterations in vital signs. Where these activities take place depends on the staffing and operational processes in the organization. Preoperative medications and regional blocks can be administered in the preoperative preparation area or in a patient hold area that is connected to the surgical suite (Fig. 1). Understanding how this part of the process will be conducted, before facility design, helps ensure appropriate and adequate spaces to support all processes.

A final issue to consider regarding the preoperative preparation area involves whether the space will be used for phase II recovery processes. Many perioperative procedure locations are limited by space. Any time a space can be used for multiple functions, the amount of space required for the entire process can be minimized. Space used for multiple functions makes good business sense. However, preoperative preparation area planning must encompass the processes to be used, to ensure patient care spaces adequate to preventing bottlenecks in patient flow when patients are bring prepared for procedures, and when they are being received after the procedure is completed, should this area also serve as phase II recovery. A planning guideline for determining the number of preoperative preparation stations is 1.5

stations per OR or procedure room [5]. As the guideline implies, clinical areas other than the operating suite may process patients through the preoperative preparation area before an invasive procedure. Processing volumes for these procedure rooms should be included in planning for the number of preoperative preparation stations needed. These planning concerns apply to ambulatory surgery centers and hospital-based services.

Operating room support areas

The OR suite has specific functions required to support the entire OR process. The first, and probably most critical to running a smooth OR suite, is the OR control area. This area is generally where staff determine the current status of all ORs, surgical patients in the OR suite, and changes to the current day's surgical schedule. This function can be assisted by manual or electronic processes. Staff involved in any phase of the perioperative process (ie, nurses, technicians, surgeons, anesthesia providers, and so forth), may physically come to this area or gain access by means of phone lines or an internal paging system. When planning the OR suite, it is critical to plan a location for the OR control area that allows accessibility to all personnel expected to interface with control functions of the OR suite. It is also important to understand all the functions that are intended to take place in this area, to allow enough space for their accomplishment. Plans for use of information technology systems should also be known, to allow for proper installation of the system and connectivity to areas that will be using such systems.

The OR suite cannot operate without the use of some type of OR surgical case scheduling system. Again, the type of scheduling process needs to be known during the planning phase of a facility, to provide the appropriate environment for the scheduler and physical and electronic access by others involved in the process. The scheduler's area should likely be near the OR suite but it may not necessarily need to be located within the semirestricted or restricted areas of the suite.

Frequently, the sizing of staff dressing rooms seems to be inadequate. When planning staff dressing rooms, realistic projections for those personnel who will need to use the dressing rooms is critical. It is easy to account for staff working in the OR suite and the surgeons who require space in the dressing rooms. The shortfall in planning

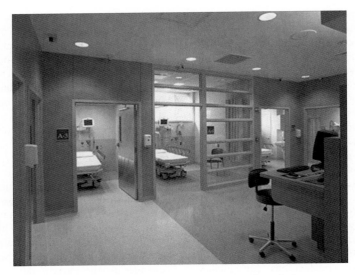

Fig. 1. Pre-operative/phase II recovery private bed.

comes when considering visitors and ancillary personnel who must change into scrub attire to access the semirestricted and restricted areas of the OR suite to assist with procedures. In addition to ancillary hospital personnel, planning for the following personnel should be considered when right-sizing the dressing rooms: surgical residents and other students; vendors who check on and order surgical supplies; educators providing presentations; adjunct surgical assistive staff for each surgical specialty; and PACU staff, if they will share dressing rooms with the OR staff. One must take the time to think about all the personnel who access the semirestricted and restricted areas of the OR and whether they need locker space in the changing rooms. Additionally, planners must be realistic about the size of lockers required. Many times in the past, half-size lockers have been programmed as a means of saving space. Some transient personnel may be able to use half-size lockers. However, it is more likely that most personnel using the dressing rooms need a locker that can accommodate a full change of clothes, space for personal valuables, and coats or jackets.

One other issue related to staff dressing rooms that must be considered is the process for distributing surgical scrubs. Some organizations use scrub attire dispensers, which allow staff to sign out surgical scrubs individually. These scrub dispensers require space and need to be included in the planning process. If scrub dispensers are not used, an area must be provided in which to store clean scrubs and dispose of soiled scrubs. These functions should not be neglected in planning the space.

Depending on the number of ORs in the surgical suite, an organization may want to consider the need for a small decontamination/sterilization function in the main OR area. Cost containment pressures sometimes limit the number of surgical specialty instruments that can be purchased. This limitation can require frequent reprocessing of specialty surgical instrumentation. Traditionally, OR suites have been built with substerile rooms containing flash sterilizers between ORs or with flash sterilizers in the sterile core area of the OR suite, where such instrumentation is flash sterilized between cases. Specialty surgical instruments may not be sent to central sterile for reprocessing between cases because of the length of turnaround time or fear of losing a costly specialty instrument. If these are concerns for an organization, planning a small decontamination area with a pass-through washer/sterilizer and a small wrap and sterilizing function should be considered, to provide optimal reprocessing of such instrumentation. Planning an area with this function may decrease or eliminate the need for substerile rooms to be programmed immediately adjacent to ORs.

OR suites are equipment-intensive areas of the hospital. OR suites are also traditionally located far away from the primary biomedical equipment maintenance section in the facility. For this reason, planning a biomedical equipment maintenance area as part of, or in close proximity to, the

OR suite may be advantageous, allowing quicker equipment maintenance processing and routine maintenance of OR equipment. Such a function could also serve other areas close to the OR, such as PACU and intensive care nursing units, both of which are also equipment-intensive areas of the hospital.

Another important function to consider when planning support areas for the OR suite is waste removal, including nonbiohazard waste, biohazard waste, soiled linen, and specimens. Waste and soiled linen repositories need to be sized adequately and located properly to allow access by the surgical suite personnel bringing waste from the ORs for transport out of the OR suite, and by housekeeping personnel who transport this waste from the OR suite out of the facility. If a facility performs a high volume of orthopedic endoscopy procedures, biohazard fluid removal may be of such volume that a fluid retrieval system is needed. Such a system may require a docking station for fluid disposal and should be planned for in the design of the OR suite. Specimen handling is mentioned here because of the frequent mishandling incidents that occur but are not necessarily reported as sentinel events in a facility. Proper labeling, logging in and out, and careful transport of specimens are critical steps when handling specimens, to ensure accurate postoperative diagnosis and treatment of surgical patients. Specimen handling areas in the OR suite should be planned with appropriate ventilation hoods for when formaldehyde or other specimen preservatives with toxic fumes are used. A specific area for logging specimens for transport from the OR to pathology services should be planned. Depending on the frequency of frozen sections performed on surgical specimens, consideration should be given to planning a space in the OR suite for pathologists to perform this function, which may allow better specimen handling and patient diagnosis.

Finally, planning staff support areas in the OR suite for conferences, education, and breaks is important. Frequently, OR suite staff needs to conduct or participate in meetings or provide educational opportunities within the OR suite, to minimize staff time away from patient care. Conferencing and education spaces need to be planned to support these functions within the OR suite. Additionally, work breaks and meal breaks are of short duration, requiring OR suite staff to stay within the confines of the department to maximize their rest periods. Appropriately sized staff break areas are needed to support the staff and allow them a restful place to take a break in what is normally a high stress area of the facility. These three functions are grouped together so that they can be designed as one multifunction area to maximize the use of space.

Equipment and supply storage for surgical suites

Surgical suites never seem to have enough equipment and supply storage areas. This perception and reality are likely due to surgical technology changes over the past 30 years, changes that will continue, which have led to the planning of support areas to accommodate service-specific equipment and supplies for certain surgical services in the surgical suite. In addition, understanding how central sterile supports the surgical suites and other procedure rooms impacts how and where sterile supply is planned in the facility.

Certain surgical services use large pieces of equipment and service-specific supplies requiring storage in the surgical suite. Open-heart surgery requires storage for the heart/lung pump. Neurosurgery has multiple large pieces of equipment, as does orthopedic surgery. Fluoroscopic and mobile radiograph equipment is used by multiple services and demands large storage spaces in the surgical suite. Specialty-specific equipment and supply storage areas that support many specialty surgical services are now a necessity and must be planned for when designing surgical support spaces. Once again, knowing who is going to be using the surgical suite is key to planning and designing appropriate support space in the surgical suite.

Storage of service-specific sterile supplies, in addition to equipment, accounts for a large footprint in the sterile storage area of the surgical suite. Every surgical service uses some type of disposable surgical supplies. Endoscopy procedures for general surgery; gynecology; orthopedics; urology; ear, nose, and throat; cardiothoracic (and the list goes on) all require specialty-specific endoscopy supplies, which, added to the suture and other required service-specific sterile supplies, increases dramatically the demand for sterile storage in the surgical suite. Just-in-time supply delivery systems help reduce the amount of space needed to store these items, but significant space is required nonetheless.

The location of central sterile and the process used to prepare supplies for surgical cases impacts how sterile storage areas are planned in the surgical suite. If central sterile is on a different floor than the surgical suites, then planning more sterile storage with the surgical suites may better suit operational needs. The use of surgical case carts for preparation and storage of surgical case supplies drives the need for additional sterile storage in the immediate area of the surgical suite. The following questions must be answered if case carts are used:

- Is central sterile stocking the surgical supplies on the carts, or is this done in conjunction with sterile supplies stocked by the surgical suite personnel?
- Are multiple surgical cases stocked on one case cart, or does every surgical case have a case cart?

Storage space must be planned for if case carts are used. The issue is where to plan the space (ie, in the surgical suite area or in central sterile). This decision is based on the processes the organization intends to use and where central sterile resides.

Once surgical cases are completed, the case carts must be returned to central sterile for processing dirty instrumentation and case cart cleaning. Adequate space must be planned, not only for the intended flow of dirty case carts from the surgical suite to the central sterile decontamination area but also for cleaning the case carts. Use of manual cleaning processes versus automatic cart cleaning machines will drive the amount of space needed for this function.

If central sterile is on a different floor and is not immediately adjacent to the surgical suite, the hours of operation for central sterile can impact the amount of sterile storage that is planned in the sterile core or cores of the surgical suite. If central sterile staff is available 24 hours per day, then the surgical suite has someone to call during evening and nighttime cases, to assist with retrieval of instruments and sterile supplies that may not be stored in the sterile core. However, if central sterile hours of operation are limited to the elective surgery hours, one may need to anticipate more storage in the sterile core for instrumentation and sterile supplies, and a shift of sterile storage space from central sterile to the sterile core. This issue of support hours for central sterile is likely to be more of a concern in a hospital-based setting, where emergency surgical cases are performed around the clock, versus an ambulatory surgery center, which has specific hours of operation.

Postanesthesia care unit: phase I recovery

The first stop for most patients after an invasive procedure is the PACU, where phase I recovery takes place. Knowing the clinical areas that will send patients to the PACU for phase I recovery after an invasive procedure will drive the number of PACU beds that are needed. A guideline for planning the number of beds is to have one bed per OR or procedure room. Patients processed through the preoperative preparation area may not necessarily require PACU services. Patients who received light sedation or have achieved the milestones to qualify for phase II recovery may bypass PACU and go right to phase II recovery. Information needed to plan the number of PACU beds is the same, whether patients are recovering in an ambulatory surgery center or a hospital-based setting.

Depending on the infection control requirements analysis for the facility, a minimum of one negative pressure isolation recovery bed will likely be needed for an ambulatory surgery center. A hospital-based setting PACU may need more than one isolation recovery bed. If the facility provides transplant services, a positive pressure recovery bed may also be needed.

Recovery of pediatric patients should also be taken into consideration when planning recovery spaces. Providing a physical and auditory separation between the adult recovery area and pediatric recovery area is beneficial for both groups of patients. In addition, creating an environment that allows parents to be present during the recovery process, when appropriate, for phases I and II recovery should be included in the planning process.

Phase II recovery

After achieving the necessary level of consciousness milestones, patients will proceed from phase I to phase II recovery. Patients continue to improve their level of consciousness in this area and most are eventually discharged from the facility out of this area. Depending on the clinical areas requiring phase II recovery services, patients may come directly from a procedure room to phase II recovery. Planning phase II recovery beds depends on knowing which clinical areas will send patients to this recovery area. In an ambulatory surgery center, all patients will likely process out of the facility through phase II recovery, which is not true of all patients in a hospital-based setting.

Planning guidelines suggest allocating two phase II recovery beds per OR or procedure room. Again, this planning guideline should be modified, based on the concept of operations for the facility being planned. If the phase II recovery area also serves as the preoperative preparation area, understanding the number of services using both functions will drive the number of beds required.

An area designed to meet the needs of pediatric patients during phase II recovery should be included for those organizations performing pediatric procedures. The area should allow children to move freely and safely while providing adequate space for one or two parents to be present with each child.

Including a nourishment center in the phase II recovery area is a must. Most patients need to demonstrate the ability to tolerate intake of fluids and food before discharge from this area. The nourishment center should be accessible to staff and family members assisting patients during this phase of the perioperative process.

The voice of experience: planning perioperative facilities

Planning health care facilities to support the perioperative process involves a thorough understanding of patient use of perioperative areas and the operational concepts to be used in the facility. The voice of experience provides valuable information to ensure the final facility supports the planned functions as intended.

Ms. Norma White from Austin, Texas, has been involved with the establishment of ambulatory surgery centers from the time of their inception. Her experience with these centers goes back to the early 1970s, when she served as the administrator for Bailey Square Surgical Center in Austin, at that time the largest free-standing surgical center in the United States. Ms. White went to Washington, DC, and spoke with the Ways and Means Committee to seek approval of Medicare reimbursement for procedures done in ambulatory surgery centers. She helped the committee understand that health care rendered to patients in the ambulatory surgery setting was equal to, or exceeded, the quality of care patients traditionally received in hospital-based surgery settings. Ultimately, she was successful in gaining approval for reimbursement of surgical procedures performed in ambulatory surgery centers.

In addition to Ms. White's political expertise, she is experienced in the planning, construction, and operation of perioperative-related areas, including those in ambulatory surgery centers. She assisted in the planning, construction, and

operation of the first PACU in the city of Austin, an eight-bed unit, at Brackenridge Hospital. She also helped plan the 18,000 square foot, seven-OR Bailey Square Surgical Center in Austin. From 1995 to 1998, she was involved in the opening and management of a new surgical and ambulatory care center in the North Austin Medical Center, consisting of 10 ORs, three endoscopy suites, and a 24-bed ambulatory care unit. She is currently the director of surgical services at the Texas Orthopedics, Sports and Rehabilitation Associates Ambulatory Surgery Center in North Austin.

When asked about the evolution of perioperative facility design and what she finds to be important in planning a facility, Ms. White stated that preadmission needs an area where the nurse is able to focus and talk in private with the patient. The preoperative area design is crucial to making a positive impression on the patient when he/she first arrives in the facility. The area should be a welcoming environment for the patient and the staff who work there. Additionally, the preoperative preparation area serves well as the phase II recovery area. A good facility design supports a circular process flow where the patient starts in the preoperative preparation area, proceeds to the OR, then to PACU, and back to the preoperative preparation/phase II recovery area (N. White, personal communication, 2007).

Ms. White also commented on sterile storage planning and the location of central sterile. One should plan enough sterile storage to meet all operational needs. Flash sterilizers within the sterile core need to be convenient to multiple ORs. Enclosed instrument set pans should be used because they allow more control in preventing contamination of instrument sets during the flash sterilization process. Regarding the central sterile location, Ms. White insists central sterile be on the same floor as the OR suites. This location facilitates transport of unexpected sterile items to the OR suites in a timely manner during surgical procedures. Also, during emergency hours when central sterile is not staffed, OR staff can more easily access sterile instruments.

When asked about the impact of technology and communications on the planning of perioperative facilities, Ms. White indicated that the most vital technology at her disposal is the fax machine. The fax is a critical timesaver in obtaining information releases from patients so that the nursing staff can obtain the medical information and studies necessary to prepare surgical charts for patients' procedures. In her view, electronic documentation programs are not inclusive enough. Most use a listing of items the nurse checks off in the record. However, many times, nurses should record additional observations, yet they do not because they get in the habit of checking items off, as opposed to adding important comments, which can be a problem if the records are reviewed for a legal issue. Ms. White also explained that the use of electronic documentation is not compatible with all procedures. For example, bilateral myringotomy tube placement takes less time than is required to log onto the computer and enter the information required in an electronic format. This example is only one of many that show how electronic documentation slows down the surgical process.

Today, facility planning for perioperative services is more complex than ever. It is imperative that the planner capture (or understand) the surgical needs of the facility so that space is allocated properly to meet the requirements of preadmissions, preoperative processing, storage, ancillary space, recovery, and staff work areas. It is essential to capture cognitively the time and space needs, based on the complexity of the caseload and recovery demands anticipated at each facility.

Well-planned and functional health care facilities are developed by involving clinical personnel in the planning stages from the very inception of the idea to build or renovate. Because of the specialized nature of the perioperative process, it is critical to have experienced perioperative personnel on the planning team to ensure that the end facility supports perioperative clinical functions. Involving perioperative personnel in facility development allows them to articulate the importance of planning perioperative support spaces that will enable staff to provide the scope of services and use the patient care processes agreed on by all members of the perioperative health care team. Space allocation and fresh perspectives on future designs are essential when planning for a facility that will be required to provide services to a community for years to come.

References

[1] Moore R. Hospitals struggle with soaring building costs. Birmingham Business Journal 2006;3:1. Available at: http://www.bizjournals.com/birmingham/stories/2006/08/28/focus3.html?t=printable. Accessed September 26, 2007.

[2] Greene J. Climbing construction cost: skyrocketing materials costs force project financing changes. Hospitals & Health Networks 2006;0611:1. Available at: http://www.hhnmag.com/hhnmag_app/jsp/articledisplay.jsp?dcrpath=HHNMAG/PubsNewsArticle/data/2006November/0611HHN_FEA_Construction&;domain=HHNMAG. Accessed September 26, 2007.

[3] Appleby J, Cauchon D. Hospital building booms in 'burbs. USA Today January 3, 2006; Available at: http://www.usatoday.com/news/health/2006-01-03-hospital-boom_x.htm. Accessed September 26, 2007.

[4] The Facility Guidelines Institute, The American Institute of Architects Academy of Architecture for Health, with assistance from the U.S. Department of Health and Human Services. Guidelines for design and construction of health care facilities. Washington, DC: The American Institute of Architects; 2006.

[5] Department of Defense, Defense Medical Facilities Office, with assistance from Rogers, Lovelock and Fritz. Department of defense medical planning criteria and medical equipment guide plates: DoD space planning criteria for health facilities. Winter Park (FL): Rogers, Lovelock and Fritz; 2002; Available at: http://199.211.83.169/ocfo/ppmd/criteria.cfm. Accessed September 26, 2007.

ELSEVIER
SAUNDERS

Perioperative Nursing Clinics 3 (2008) 63–72

PERIOPERATIVE
NURSING
CLINICS

Alternative Waste Management Strategies

George F. Nussbaum, PhD, RN, CNOR

Graduate School of Nursing, Perioperative Clinical Nurse Specialist Program, Uniformed Services University,
4301 Jones Bridge Road, Bethesda, MD 20814, USA

Waste management is an invisible part of the daily activities in a busy operating room. Although most everyone can agree that the control of the various forms of waste and the confusing definitions, regulatory compliances, and local policies are costly, little has been done to conceptualize the magnitude, complexity, and economic impact of the issue (Fig. 1).

A handwritten sign on a waste collector's large collection cart in a large teaching facility reads, "No one knows what I do until I don't do it." He may well have a key to the solution. If, in fact, he "stopped doing it" and a study was conducted on the waste being generated, beginning with the outside supply vendor all the way to the final disposal location, the results would serve to illustrate graphically the magnitude of the issue. The analysis of the issue does not start with the waste collector; it begins at the point of product purchase [1]. Waste minimization starts with reducing or eliminating it at the source. The most effective solutions can found by analyzing the multiple non–value-added processes, steps, and wasted personnel efforts that are significantly contributing to the problem throughout the facility. Begin with a careful analysis of surgically related products that enter the facility and then an inventory of all the purchased items that leave as a form of waste. Analyze the numbers of personnel required to order, manage an order, load materials, transfer and unload, stock in a warehouse, break down to the unit of issue, and discard cardboard containers. Calculate the number of times and the number of personnel required to transport these items to the point of use and the

volumes of waste in the form of wrappers and containers collected.

Over the past $3\frac{1}{2}$ decades, changes in surgical health care delivery have radically altered the types of instrumentation and surgical products that are routinely used. We moved from an exclusively nondisposable environment to one that is predominantly disposable, with the exception of the durable surgical instrument sets. In the continuing and growing efforts for minimally invasive procedures, industry leads the way in the production of disposable products that provide the portals through which these procedures are accomplished. Along with disposable surgical instrumentation, the full range of sterile surgical attire and draping materials has evolved. With this has been a full shift in the generation, types, and disposition of the waste generated by surgical procedures [1].

Categorically, these include the following:

- Surgical patient drapes
- Surgical table, ring stand, and Mayo drapes
- Surgical gowns
- Sterile team gloves
- Sterile durable instrument sets
- Sterile basins
- Disposable items (eg, blades, suture) and instruments (eg, trocars, miscellaneous portals and graspers, scissors)
- All types of surgical sponges and packing
- Nonsterile bed linen, blankets, pillowcases, positioning aids, and pressure prevention aids
- Suction bottles containing the waste from anesthesia-generated secretions and surgical wound residue and irrigation

In 1967, none of the items listed were disposable. Every item in the operating room was sent to the hospital laundry or to the sterile processing

E-mail address: nussbaumgf@verizon.net

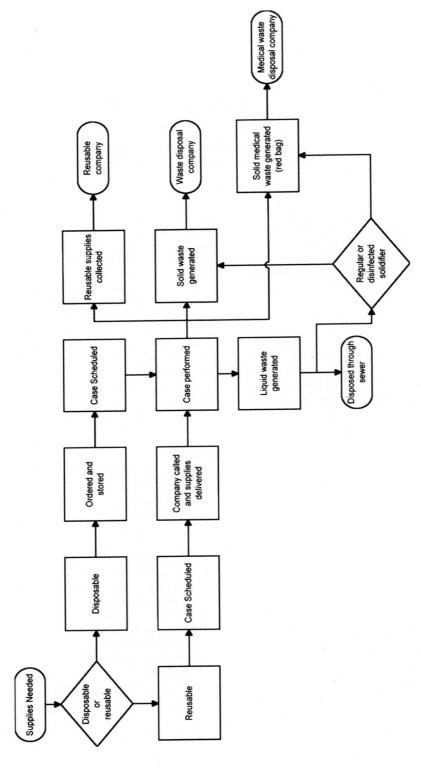

Fig. 1. Surgical waste stream.

department. The amount of material sent out as waste was minimal. In 2007, virtually everything, with the exception of durable instruments, is discarded as waste in some form. Between 2 and 4 million tons of hospital waste are generated and discarded annually from health care facilities alone [2]. Clearly, there have been advances in technology and surgical practices. New threats have been introduced that were not known or present in the days of complete nondisposable equipment, including HIV, hepatitis B, hepatitis C, methicillin-resistant *Staphylococcus aureus* (MRSA), vancomycin-resistant *Enterococcus* (VRE), Creutzfeldt-Jacob disease (CJD), *Acinetobacter*, severe acute respiratory syndrome (SARS), and other viruses that threaten to inflict disease on health care personnel and patients [3]. Reactions to these new threats appeared in the form of universal precaution standards and the Medical Waste Tracking Act (1988) [4]. By this time, disposable use was the norm and the natural tendency was to treat everything as infectious waste and send it to the incinerator. Economic and environmental variables soon joined the equation. The requirement to do it faster, better, less costly, and environmentally safe became the expectation.

The operating room is typically considered a cost-generating area. The fact that it is also one of the largest and most costly waste-generating areas is overlooked in most institutions. That waste, from a cost and published review perspective, should be less than 15% regulated medical waste (RMW) or "red bag waste." The remainder of the waste generated in the operating room in the form of solid waste or regular trash should comprise the remainder. From a typical cost perspective, red bag waste costs a facility 10 to 25 times the cost of solid waste [5]. The amount of waste generated daily in every business and organization in the United Sates is staggering compared with European nations. We have disposable containers, boxes, and paper and plastic bags for everything imaginable. A food court in a typical shopping mall requires one or more full-time personnel to manage waste containers. Health care facilities are no exception, with the added problem of the confusion as to what might be potentially infectious. Up to 85% of waste that should be disposed as solid waste is instead placed in infectious waste containers [5,6].

Waste cost estimates

The economics for disposition of hospital-generated waste is driven by multiple variables, including the weight and volume; the locale; crossing state lines; and regulatory interpretations by local, state, and federal mandates. The following are the current ranges available from published reports and unstructured surveys:

$0.02 to $0.06 per pound for solid waste
$0.30 to $1.25 per pound for biohazardous/ infectious waste (red bag)
$1.00 to $6.00 per pound for hazardous waste

Medical waste defined

In the course of treating patients, hospital personnel generate a remarkable amount of waste. By classification, multiple categories of wastes are created, including RMW, also referred to as infectious waste; hazardous chemical waste; and recyclable, reusable, and solid waste. Within these categories are further classifications, including liquids and sharp items (Fig. 2).

There is not a universally accepted definition for RMW; however, the definitions offered by regulatory agencies are similar. The Environmental Protection Agency (EPA), the Centers for Disease Control and Prevention (CDC), the World Health Organization (WHO), and the Occupational Safety and Health Administration (OSHA) agree that "regulated medical waste includes those wastes with the potential for causing infection and for which special precautions are prudent" [7].

The CDC's guidance for Universal Precautions suggests that blood and body fluid precautions be used for all patients regardless of their infection status. These precautions stem mainly from the need to minimize exposure to the viruses and microbial organisms responsible for causing disease. "In effect, all free flowing blood, blood products, body fluids containing visible blood, and other specific body fluids such as cerebrospinal fluid, synovial fluid, pleural fluid, peritoneal fluid, pericardial fluid, amniotic fluid, vaginal secretions, and semen should be handled with universal precautions and managed as regulated medical waste" [7–9]. All 50 states have specific regulations that address medical waste. These regulations are extremely diverse and vary from simple definitions to stringent treatment, storage, and disposal requirements [7]. Several states stipulate that sharps must be rendered unrecognizable (defined as less than 0.5 inch in length) before final disposal.

The EPA defines infectious waste in the *Guide for Infectious Waste Management (EPA530-SW-86-014)* as waste that "contains pathogens with

WASTE STREAMS

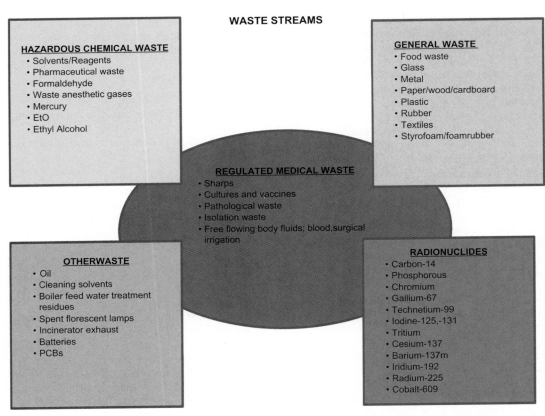

HAZARDOUS CHEMICAL WASTE
- Solvents/Reagents
- Pharmaceutical waste
- Formaldehyde
- Waste anesthetic gases
- Mercury
- EtO
- Ethyl Alcohol

GENERAL WASTE
- Food waste
- Glass
- Metal
- Paper/wood/cardboard
- Plastic
- Rubber
- Textiles
- Styrofoam/foamrubber

REGULATED MEDICAL WASTE
- Sharps
- Cultures and vaccines
- Pathological waste
- Isolation waste
- Free flowing body fluids; blood,surgical irrigation

OTHERWASTE
- Oil
- Cleaning solvents
- Boiler feed water treatment residues
- Spent florescent lamps
- Incinerator exhaust
- Batteries
- PCBs

RADIONUCLIDES
- Carbon-14
- Phosphorous
- Chromium
- Gallium-67
- Technetium-99
- Iodine-125,-131
- Tritium
- Cesium-137
- Barium-137m
- Iridium-192
- Radium-225
- Cobalt-609

Fig. 2. US Army Center for Health and Promotion and Preventive Medicine. A commander's guide to regulated medical waste management at army medical treatment facilities. Available at: http://chppm-www.apgea.army.mil/documents/TG/TECHGUID/TG177.pdf. (*Adapted from* US Army Center for Health and Promotion and Preventive Medicine. A commander's guide to regulated medical waste management at Army medical treatment facilities. TG 177. Aberdeen Proving Ground, MD: US Army; 2001. Available at: http://chppm-www.apgea.army.mil/documents/TG/TECHGUID/TG177.pdf.)

sufficient virulence and quantity so that exposure to the waste by a susceptible host could result in an infectious disease" [8]. Included in this reference as RMW are blood-soaked bandages, discarded surgical gloves, discarded surgical instruments, needles, removed body organs, and discarded lancets [8]. Most medical wastes do not meet these criteria.

A common confusion point is the requirement and interpretation by states that waste is considered RMW if it contains free-flowing blood or fluids or materials like sponges and lap packs saturated with blood, bloody fluid, or caked blood. This OSHA rule defines RMW but does not regulate medical waste disposal. This definition has been used by many states and facilities to determine waste classification policies. Many facilities prefer to err on the side of caution, partly in fear of a large fine or incident involving real or perceived risk to waste management personnel [10,11].

Appropriate disposal policies for all waste streams need to address worker safety, public health, and environmental considerations in addition to regulatory compliance. After several decades of disposable use, there is a need for a dramatic cultural shift to consider disposal technologies and services as part of a renewed waste management concept. This system requires a change in thinking about upstream waste management, including the elimination or minimization of some of the wastes and reuse and recycling of others [10]. By definition, infectious waste is that fraction of medical waste that has the real potential to transmit an infectious disease. According to most authorities, infectious waste should not exceed 15% of the total hospital waste stream [12]. Recent published studies indicate that essentially everything generated in the operating room as waste leaves the facility as RMW rather than being carefully screened and separated [6].

The prevention of disease transmission to patients or to health care personnel is the primary intent of infectious waste management. The emphasis requires starts on the management of the process rather than technologic fixes supplied by industry. Many times, this has proved to be an expensive diversion rather than an effective solution [12].

Goals for the management of all health care facility–generated waste should include the following:

- Reduce or eliminate it.
- Contain costs associated with waste.
- Understand the true categories and definitions of waste.
- Appreciate waste as a "non–value-added" component of the surgical process so that it can be systematically analyzed and functionally approached.
- Establish an environment in the perioperative setting that is safe from physical and health hazards for staff and patients.
- Reduce all risks for occupational illnesses and injuries.
- Consideration of the long-term effects of surgically generated waste, beginning with the acquisition of the surgical supplies through the ultimate disposition of all waste, on the environment, people, equipment, and property.
- Remain fully compliant with all regulations imposed by federal, state, and local laws. It is important to note that the requirements of some states for the management of RMW exceed those of other states.
- Maintain constant vigilance and an education process covering the range of personnel from the purchasing agent to the landfill contractor regarding the risks associated with hazardous and infectious waste.
- Establish flawless administrative and engineering controls to create, sustain, and maintain safe work practices [13].

A frequently cited study using the collected waste from 27 surgical procedures consisting of spinal, cardiovascular, orthopedic, and general surgery generating 610.5 lb (274.4 kg) illustrates the issues. The contents by weight consisted of disposable linen (39%), paper (7%), plastic (23%), and miscellaneous (27%). The contents by volume consisted of disposable linen and plastic (69%), plastic basins (23%), and miscellaneous (7%). The researchers intentionally did not include the weight or the contents of body fluids containers in suction canisters. Linen, paper, and recyclable paper accounted for 73% by weight and 93% by volume. The study concluded that a 73% reduction in weight and 93% by volume could be realized if reusable products were substituted for the items disposed [14].

A similar recently published report illustrates a continued practice of expensive waste management. In this study, 92% of the weight of red bag waste was discarded inappropriately as biohazardous waste [15]. These reports signal the need to examine current practices critically with respect to all waste generated in the perioperative environment from the multiple perspectives of cost and personnel resource requirements from purchasing through final disposition, recycle, or reuse procedures.

Cost estimates are as follows:

$0.02 to $0.06 for normal waste
$0.19 to $0.40 for biohazardous waste
$1.00 to $6.00 for hazardous waste

Medical wastes as facility space issues

Waste management has an impact on facility space requirements. There is a necessity for locations to separate the various types of waste at the site of origin and another requisite for staging disposal locations, such as a loading dock or a logistic warehouse space. There must be appropriate areas to wash and clean utility vehicles that transport soiled materials within the facility and locations to store clean and soiled utility vehicles. There needs to be ample space for soiled and clean utility rooms that are readily accessible by transportation personnel away from the public thoroughfares and public elevators if possible.

The systems selected for management of waste need to be compatible with and included in design and construction projects during the planning phases of a project rather than as an afterthought. Waste is not glamorous and is seldom considered, but the cost and safety factors are staggering. The flow of materials into and the waste flow that leaves the entire perioperative area need to be planned into the physical layout in any renovation or new construction project. Failure to consider the traffic flow patterns and locations for these items results in built-in inefficiencies. The full cradle-to-grave process must be considered for everything that enters the perioperative environment and requires some form of final disposition. This includes waste anesthetic gasses (WAG), smoke plume, specimens, sharps, instruments, loaner sets, disposable and nondisposable sterile items, recyclable paper, plastic items, liquid waste, and linens.

Reconsideration of nondisposable solutions

Shaner and McRae [12] propose that "facilities should firmly support the judicious reuse of materials and should explore opportunities where the use of reprocessed materials is feasible and available." This effort within hospitals should provide quality products and thwart efforts to increase reliance on disposables. Disposables are costly, increase waste generation, and have not demonstrated definitive decreases in infection rates in the perioperative arena.

Liquid waste

Liquid regulated medical waste disposal options

Liquid waste generated during surgical procedures can be disposed using one of four methods (Fig. 3):

- Close the system, secure the top and ports on the canister (container), and place the contents in a red bag as infectious waste. This is the least favorable option. The contents are subject to leaking if the lids or ports dislodge, potentially exposing waste management workers as the liquid waste is transferred and transported to the final destination. The

liquid contents in a 3-L canister weigh 7.5 lb. Estimates per pound vary by state and location. Costs range from $0.60 to greater than $1.00 per canister.

- Transport the filled canisters to a soiled utility area, and pour the contents in a hopper utility sink into the normal waste water system. No formal research data are published indicating the prevalence of this practice; however, industry estimates are that from 30% to greater than 65% of facilities discard liquid surgical waste in this manner. This is the most economic practice for health care facilities and the one with the highest potential risks to staff and patients. Full personal protective equipment (PPE) is required while pouring the contents of liquid surgical waste. Normal practice suggests that gowns and gloves be removed before leaving the operating room by scrubbed personnel. This would require donning a new gown, gloves, and mask if the operating room staff is responsible for discarding waste at the completion of a procedure. This sets up discretionary PPE use negating safety, engineering controls, and compliance during operating room turnover.
- A 2006 survey of 340 members of the Association of Occupational Health Professionals (AOHP) in health care revealed the three most significant concerns for health care workers to be safe patient handling, blood-borne pathogen exposure,

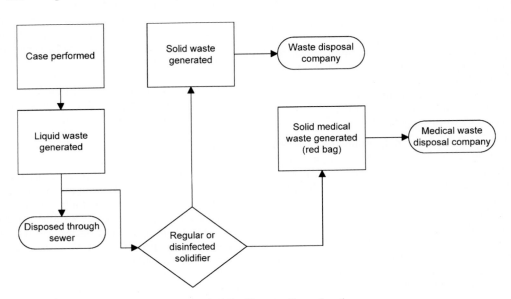

Fig. 3. Surgical liquid waste disposal options.

and respiratory protection. A total of 73.5% of those surveyed were specifically concerned about the exposure to blood and liquid waste [16].

- The next alternative method involves adding a solidifying agent to the container to create a solid gelatinous mass. This eliminates the potential for fluid leakage but does not reduce the weight of the canister as RMW. A supplemental practice is the addition of sanitizing agents, including chlorine or glutaraldehyde. In some locations, states tolerate this as "treated" medical waste and allow the canister and contents to be disposed as solid waste (white bag). There are limited data supporting the safety and efficacy of this practice.
- Recently introduced are closed disposal systems. These are self-contained units that collect fluid waste at the surgical field and allow for disposition directly into the waste water system using hands-free and no-exposure methods.

The primary advantages of these systems include the following:

- Minimize risk to staff by minimizing the number of times and the number of personnel required to handle the liquid waste.
- Reduce RMW and RMW transportation.
- Eliminate bulk weight and volume leaving the facility.

It should be noted that all states, with the exception of the District of Columbia, allow this practice.

No matter how you view it, RMW is expensive. Priorities should be protection of staff and patients, costs associated with practices, and environmental concerns [17].

Workers who handle waste tend to be the lowest paid and the least educated members in the health care setting. These personnel often become unseen and not considered with respect to proper instruction in the proper handling of various wastes generated in a facility. Severe fines occur when personnel are exposed to harmful wastes or wastes are disposed improperly by regulating agencies (Tables 1 and 2) [12].

Human blood and blood products

Because it is impractical to test all blood for the presence of every possible pathogen, it is prudent to manage all blood and blood products as infectious waste. It is logical to extend this practice to the wastes associated with blood specimens and to handle them as though they

Table 1
Fluid medical waste solidifiers

Colby manufacturing corporations	ViraSorb[a]
DeRoyal Industries[a]	DeRoyal Solidifier
DiSorb Systems, Inc.[b]	SafeSorb
Metrex, Inc.[c]	PremCide
	Canister Express
	The Solidifier
Microtek Medical, Inc.[d]	LTS Plus
	Isosorb
Safetec of America, Inc.[e]	Red-Z
	Green-Z
	Yellow-Z
Zapatec LLC[f]	Zaploc

[a] Powell, Tennessee.
[b] Philadelphia, Pennsylvania.
[c] Orange, California.
[d] Columbus, Missouri.
[e] Greensboro NC Inc., Buffalo, New York.
[f] McLeansville, North Carolina.

were contaminated. Two recommended treatment methods are steam sterilization and incineration. In addition, blood and blood products may be discharged directly to a sanitary sewer for treatment in the municipal sewerage treatment system provided that secondary treatment is available [18].

Table 2
Surgical fluid waste collection and disposal systems

Company	Product
Bemis[a]	Vac-U-Port
	Vac-U-Station
	Quick Drain
Cardinal[b]	Medi-Vac
	SAF-T-Pump
DeRoyal Industries[c]	Aqua-Box
Dornach Medical Systems[d]	Transposal
Merit Medical Systems, Inc.[e]	Merit Disposal
MD Technologies[f]	Environ-mate DM 6000 Series
	Suction Drain System
Stryker Medical[g]	Neptune

[a] Sheboygan, Wisconsin.
[b] Dublin, Ohio.
[c] Powell, Tennessee.
[d] St. Louis, Missouri.
[e] South Jordan, Utah.
[f] Galena, Illinois.
[g] Kalamazoo, Michigan.

Surgical linen and drapes

Waste generation is directly related to purchasing and supply practices and habits. A generation of perioperative nurses has only known the use of nonreprocessible, single-use, sterile surgical products. Many of today's seasoned operating room supervisors can remember nondisposable gowns, table covers, and draping material, with the associated labor of light tables, folding rooms, and iron-on patches [12,15]. Many debates and discussions were conducted in Association of periOperative Registered Nurses (AORN) forums with respect to the number of allowable patches per item, thread counts in cotton muslin products, and other issues related to suitability for use in surgical settings. Light tables, folding tables, and lint became history with the introduction of disposable packs. Manufacturers soon learned the art of marketing custom packs with every conceivable item being "built" into a single bundle, with the promise of cost savings in time, effort, and efficiency. The savings that were to be realized from fewer Central Sterile personnel quickly evaporated with the new requirement for waste management personnel and additional expensive locations to hold waste awaiting removal.

In the early 1990s, new nondisposable surgical gowns were introduced to the market; however, without staff, hospitals were no longer equipped or staffed to launder, inspect, fold, and sterilize surgical drapes and gowns. Most operating room supervisors, cognizant of muslin gowns and drapes, were not the least bit interested in revisiting those issues. The introduction of the disposable custom packs was a more than satisfactory solution. For a time AMSCO Sterilizer Company (STERIS, Mentor, Ohio) initiated plants throughout the country to provide nondisposable solutions in the way of sterile reprocessed drapes, gowns, and table and Mayo stand covers without winning the hearts and minds of those remembering the not so "good old days" of muslin. Ultimately, the AMSCO Sterilizer Company product and services were acquired by Sterile Recovery, Inc. (SRI, Elkridge, Maryland). SRI has the largest US Food and Drug Administration (FDA)–approved reprocessing centers in the United States. The American Hospital Association reports 5747 registered hospitals in the United States [19]. SRI reports having 275 hospitals that use sterile nondisposable packs consisting of gowns, towels, back table covers, Mayo stand covers, and drapes. The company also reports 371 hospitals that use sterile nondisposable basin sets. Individual items currently being supplied in disposable custom packs, such as surgical sponges, Ascepto syringes, and suction tubing, are supplied by SRI with the nondisposable gown and drape pack. The disposable products are custom selected by individual customers and sterilized as a single unit, eliminating the need to open each item. Changes to the content of these disposable items can be easily altered without having to exhaust a 6-month supply of custom surgical drape packs currently provided by other vendors. Hospitals that use reprocessible surgical gowns and drapes, for example, do so under a service rather than a purchase contract. The service includes the supply of the sterile product from an FDA-regulated facility; the retrieval of the used product; and the return transport, laundering, inspecting, folding, and sterilizing of the items for reuse. This service is becoming available as an addition to primary vendor contracts for those facilities wishing to change to nondisposable use items but not wanting to lose the benefit of existing economic purchasing agreements.

A study published in 2001 in Denmark concluded an overall equal rating with respect to comfort and barrier protection between disposable and reusable surgical gowns. Both products have an environmental impact as waste or water consumption; however, in this study and location, with the reusable products tested in best and worst scenarios, the reprocessible products were slightly superior [20].

Two studies, one conducted in Germany and the other in the United States, concluded that there are no conclusive arguments to support a clinical superiority between disposable gowns and drapes and the reuse components. Both studies clearly establish that disposables generate a considerable amount of clinical waste [21].

Comparative studies conducted in the United States by manufacturers of disposable surgical supplies are inconclusive with respect to the superiority of disposable or nondisposable products. Dated studies comparing reuse and disposable products have limited relevance because of poor study design and the introduction of product improvements and efficiencies in water and power conservation strategies [9]. The use of reprocessible drapes, gowns, table coverings, and basins can reduce the weight and volume of surgical waste by greater than 75% [14].

Research opportunities

There are no significant qualitative or quantitative research methodologies or designs currently available to define all the issues associated with biohazardous waste materials. The few studies available are biased by vendors toward the sale of disposable custom products or reuse products. Approaches like those demonstrated by the Lean and six Sigma strategies [22] provide tools by which the relative value, or nonvalue, in processes can be analyzed and suitable measurement strategies can be applied. Appropriately designed research using validated methodologic approaches can lead to data on which sound decisions contrasting alternative solutions in the disposable, reuse, and recycle matrix for liquid waste; gowns, drapes, and table coverings; basin ware; and appropriate terminal disposition processes can be selected.

Research needs to focus on product space requirements, purchasing practices, costs for use and disposition, inventory, storage, multiple transfer activities between locations, impact on the room turnover process, impact on personnel requirements, and safety. The application of appropriate study designs and methodologies should focus on a 20/20 vision for the future and make sound economic decisions for the protection of staff, patients, and environment and financial resources.

Health care professionals should engage independent experts in study design, methodologic rigor, and appropriate statistical tools to create and validate publishable and replicable evidence to support sound clinical decisions. These studies should contrast alternative products on the basis of the following:

- Life cycle costs, which involves the process of obtaining, transferring, using, and disposing of the product
- Personnel requirements associated with these processes
- Personnel satisfaction with the products and process
- Personnel safety and compliance with EPA environmental controls
- Facility liability costs for noncompliance along the product life cycle continuum

Summary

The health care industry and, more specifically, the perioperative setting have a 30-year history of acquiring a complete disposable habit. The relatively inexpensive costs of incineration of all waste provided an economic incentive for facilities to downsize personnel required to manage durable goods. That philosophy was sustainable and encouraged by the manufacturers of disposable sterile products. This past decade of these practices has resulted in dioxin and mercury emissions into the environment that are unacceptable. Incinerators are closing or being fined heavily for safety violations. Alternative and more expensive methods of waste disposal, specifically infectious and hazardous waste disposal, are driving cost upward at a rapid rate.

The fast-paced nature of perioperative nursing allows little time to contemplate the costs or impact of these practices; however, nurses are increasingly aware and concerned for their own safety and the safety of those who may be exposed to potential disease-causing materials. It seems to be the time to reconsider the benefits and liabilities of our practice habits. In many instances, handling infectious materials less or not at all may have tremendous advantages that outweigh the simple economics involved. There may be a better balance in our practice. If a concept seems promising, it should be pursued with real research. In the absence of definitive, conclusive, and compelling unbiased scientific evidence, we are directed by industry rather than by our own profession.

References

[1] Melamed A. Environmental accountability in perioperative settings. AORN J 2003;77(6):1157–68.
[2] AORN guidance statement: environmental responsibility. In: Standards, recommended practices, and guidelines. Denver (CO): AORN, Inc.; 2007. p. 251–8.
[3] Medical waste: the issue. Available at: http://www.noharm.org/us/medicalwaste/issue. Accessed October 20, 2007.
[4] Rutala WA, Mayhall CG. Medical waste. Infect Control Hosp Epidemiol 1992;13:38–48.
[5] Shaner H, McRae G. Invisible costs/visible savings: innovations in waste management for hospitals. The Nightingale Institute for Health and the Environment. Available at: http://www.nihe.org/invis.html. Accessed October 2, 2007.
[6] Laustsen G. Reduce-recycle-reuse: guidelines for promoting perioperative waste management. AORN J 2007;85:717–27.
[7] A commander's guide to regulated medical waste management; TG 177. September 2001. Available at: http://chppm-www.apgea.army.mil/documents/TG/TECHGUID/TG177.pdf. Accessed October 1, 2007.

[8] Medical waste; US EPA. Available at: http://epa. gov/epaoswer/other/medical. Accessed October 2, 2007.

[9] Rutala WA, Weber D. A review of single-use and reusable gowns and drapes in health care. Infect Control Hosp Epidemiol 2001;22:248–57.

[10] Emmanuel J. Medical waste treatment technologies: evaluating non-incineration alternatives. Healthcare without harm; 2000. Available at: http://www. noharm.org. Accessed October 1, 2007.

[11] OSHA. Occupational exposure to bloodborne pathogens. Occupational Safety and Health Administration Standard. In: 29 CFR Part 1910.1030. Available at: http://www.osha.gov/pls/oshaweb/ owadisp.show_document?p_table = STANDARDS& p_id = 10051. Accessed October 19, 2007.

[12] Shaner H, McRae G. Eleven recommendations for improving medical waste management. The Nightingale Institute for Health and the Environment. Available at: http://www.nihe.org/elevreng.html. Accessed October 3, 2007.

[13] Hazardous materials and waste management plan. Available at: http://chppm-apeagea.army.mil/IHMSM/ ms/documents/HazardousMaterialsandwaste.doc. Accessed October 2, 2007.

[14] Tieszen ME, Gruenberg JC. A quantitative, qualitative and critical assessment of surgical waste: surgeons venture through the trash can. JAMA 1992;267(20):2765–8.

[15] Lausten G. Reduce—recycle—reuse: guidelines for promoting perioperative waste management. AORN J 2007;85(4):717–27.

[16] Maheux D. A risky business. Infection control today. Available: http://www.infectioncontroltoday.com. Accessed October 20, 2007.

[17] Barlow RD. Proper liquid waste disposal mines solid gold bottom line. Healthcare Purchasing News June 2004.

[18] U.S. Environmental Protection Agency. Regulations for hazardous waste management. In: Code of Federal Regulations, 40 CFR 260-271 and 122-124. Washington, DC: U.S. Government printing Office; 1985.

[19] Available at: http://www.aha.org/resource-center/ Statistics-and-Studies/fast-facts.html. Accessed October 20, 2007.

[20] Life cycle assessment study, options for reduced impact on the environment; the environmental case of surgical gowns. European Textile Services Association; 2001.

[21] Dettenkofer M, Griesshammer R, Scherrer M, et al. [Life-cycle assessment of single-use versus reusable surgical drapes (cellulose/polyethylene–mix cotton system)]. Chirurg 1999;70(4):485–92 [In German].

[22] George ML. Lean 6 sigma for service: how to use lean speed and six sigma quality to improve services and transitions. New York: McGraw-Hill; 2003.

ELSEVIER
SAUNDERS

PERIOPERATIVE
NURSING
CLINICS

Perioperative Nursing Clinics 3 (2008) 73–84

Perioperative Staff Resiliency During Times of War and Natural Disasters

Elizabeth A.P. Vane, LTC, AN, RN, MS, CNOR[a,*],
Mary S. Hull, LTC, AN, RN, MS, PMH-NP[b,c]

[a]Department of Nursing, Perioperative Nursing Services, Landstuhl Regional Medical Center, CMR 402, APO, AE 09180, Germany
[b]Department of Nursing, Inpatient Psychiatry, Landstuhl Regional Medical Center, CMR 402, APO, AE 09180, Germany
[c]Fitness Team, 254th Combat Stress Control Detachment, Miesau, Germany

Perioperative nurses are known for their caring and their advocacy of patients who are unable to participate actively in self-care once anesthetized or sedated. Perioperative nurses provide a safe environment of care by confirming the patient's identity, verifying operative procedures, and verifying surgical sites and laterality. Perioperative nurses are responsible for patient positioning for the best surgical views and for ensuring that sterile instruments and supplies are available for use during surgery. They maintain all traffic patterns and control of all personnel in the operating room suite during surgery. Additionally, nurses in this specialty area are responsible for managing and monitoring the care not only within the surgical suite itself but throughout the entire surgical process, including interventions such as patient education, pain control, and transfer to the recovery room. Perioperative nurses must provide competent and ethical care while maintaining the privacy and dignity of every patient [1]. Culturally sensitive nursing care must be delivered in accordance with the patient's value system. Perioperative nurses need a breadth of knowledge about potentially hazardous clinical environments, including electric, thermal, laser, and radiologic energy sources; all manner of chemicals used in medications, cements,

dyes, and solutions; various devices such as powered instruments, tourniquets, and positioning devices; biologic pathogens and drug-resistant organisms; and the human factors of staffing patterns and communication strategies [1]. Perioperative staff daily stressors include frequently changing technology, intimidating management styles, multitasking, fatigue, a blaming culture, time pressure and constraints, inadequate communication among interdisciplinary groups, and patient characteristics that require unusual setups [1]. Perioperative nursing is a caring art and a science, based on the creative application of critical knowledge and skill, and the knowledge that each perioperative nurse is competent in providing quality and individualized patient care [1]. Perioperative nurses take pride in caring for others but do they realize the importance of taking care of themselves and taking care of each other?

This article describes the current interpersonal, environmental, and physical stressors for perioperative nurses who provide surgical care for patients with traumatic war injuries or those injured in natural disasters, at three echelons of care within the available health care systems. The article also describes coping strategies that lead to individual resiliency, staff resiliency, and effective teamwork, versus ineffective coping, stress-induced reactions, and maladaptive responses.

Stressors

Coping strategies

Perioperative nurses in the contemporary military environment encounter high demands

The views expressed in this article are those of the authors and do not reflect the official policy or position of the Department of the Army, the Department of Defense, or the US Government.

* Corresponding author.

E-mail address: elizabeth.vane@us.army.mil (E.A.P. Vane).

and extreme challenges on a daily basis. The surgical workload that has existed for most military and federal hospitals since 2002 involves a chaotic mix of polytrauma war-related surgeries and various peacetime and routine surgeries. The exposure to these difficult conditions and stressors, which are far outside the usual and expected workplace experience, places nurses at risk for stress reactions and responses. The same applies to perioperative nurses who respond to the chaos and turbulence brought on by natural disasters.

Interpersonal stressors

The military perioperative nursing staff consist of registered nurses and operating room technicians who work in the operating room and in the sterilization processing department. These staff members come from tri-service cultures, including active-duty members serving with the US Army, Air Force, and Navy. They are accustomed to a lifestyle of moving around the world every 2 to 4 years to fill various assignments, and thus, they usually adapt readily to new physical surroundings. The stressors they frequently encounter include registering children in new schools with various paperwork or immunizations required; registering cars and other vehicles in different states or countries; finding a new church to attend; finding new youth groups for family members to join; dealing with packing and unpacking and organizing households with available furnishings; experiencing family separations due to deployments; and working frequently with new bosses and leadership, all of whom have different expectations and priorities.

Other staff members on the team serve in the tri-service culture as reservists and have been called on to augment or backfill in various assignments. The call-up or mobilization can last from several months or longer, depending on the circumstances. From 1998 to 2002, activated reservists were called on to serve up to 180 consecutive days, which was culturally a shock to them because they had been used to serving at most 14 days in that role. That paradigm shift caused significant stressors for many reservists. Currently, reservists serve in the military treatment facilities for 1 year at a time, and that may increase to 15 months or more to match the serving time of the active-duty staff. The stressors they frequently encounter include leaving their civilian jobs to work in a military environment, hopefully in a career field in which they have the skills to perform; leaving their families behind to work with a complete group of strangers; filling in as "worker bees" in their new roles when they had been managers and supervisors in their civilian roles; needing to conform to physical stamina tests, weapons tests, uniform and grooming standards, and shift work schedules that can seem unfamiliar and daunting; working with equipment and supplies that may be unfamiliar to them; working in both the operating room and sterile processing departments; and working for much younger and less experienced active-duty counterparts. Reservists who work on active duty for less than 1 year can feel that, just as they are feeling comfortable with the active-duty roles, they complete their military obligations and must transition back to their civilian lives.

The third group consists of registered nurses and technicians from the civilian community who work in military treatment facilities as part of the nondeployed workforce. They are often the pillars who maintain the hospital's historical way of doing business, and they hold the institutional knowledge concerning many things during high turbulence and turnover of military staff. The civilian staff members may stay in the same area for many years at a time, often completing a full career in one location. The stressors they frequently encounter include having the loyalty, dedication, and "ownership" of working at that location long term and feeling as though others are not invested (because they are just passing through); potentially hitting a glass ceiling regarding promotion to leadership positions because these are usually held by the active-duty population; working for a new boss every 2 to 4 years who might be younger and less experienced than they are; seeing many staff members come and go and still supporting all the department parties and social functions; and teaching and reteaching the same skills or subjects to what can seem like a never-ending stream of workers.

All these staff members bring different skill sets, job experiences, and work expectations with them. Some will be "marathon runners" and continue in the same job for long periods of time. Other team members will be "sprinters" whose work and contributions are for the short term. But the common thread binding all members of the team is the need for stress management while balancing various personnel issues with the heavy workload that involves a mix of war-related and peacetime surgeries.

US Army perioperative nurses take pride in their ability to "conserve the fighting strength," to "get the job done," to give "selfless service from the heart," and to show "service through mobility." This attitude is great, especially when the signs and symptoms of fatigue can be recognized and dealt with so as not to cause any detriment to the mission at hand. During times of constant workload, it would be best to remember that "health care organizations, for their part, should assume responsibility for reforming work practices and for changing attitudes toward work so that exhaustion is considered as posing an unacceptable risk rather than as a sign of dedication" [2].

Signs and symptoms of fatigue include forgetfulness, poor decision making, slowed reaction time, reduced vigilance, and poor communication. Other signs include becoming fixated, apathetic, or lethargic; being in a bad mood; and nodding off [3].

Nurses who respond to natural disasters are also faced with diverse and complex challenges that stem from similar conditions. Well-meaning responders from various backgrounds may converge at the natural disaster sight with different thoughts and ideas about how things should be done. Lack of supplies, clean water, electricity, sewage processing, shelter, and roads, all can lead to the same complex challenges faced by those in a wartime setting.

Environmental stressors

Wartime nursing involves flexibility and adaptation to unfamiliar environments [4]. The same type of adjustment is required for responding to natural disasters.

"Shift work, crossing time zones, long hours of staying awake, inability to sleep in the daytime with ambient temperatures of 130 degrees F, and sleep loss accumulation can cause fatigue for those performing medical tasks and procedures" [5].

Echelons of care

Care can be provided to Department of Defense and Coalition war fighters, or to natural disaster survivors, in various settings and locations. Within each location, the level of care rendered is determined by the location of the facility with respect to the battlefield or site of the natural disaster.

Military perioperative nursing support provided to Department of Defense and Coalition war fighters can be categorized by the setting. For the purposes of this article, the term "deployed nurses" refers to those who provide services in Iraq and Afghanistan. This setting is concerned with saving life, limb, and eyesight. "Forward nurses" are those who provide services at the military medical center in Germany. This setting is concerned with the stabilization of patients for aeromedical evacuation back to the United States within 48 to 72 hours. "Stateside nurses" are perioperative nurses who participate in ongoing restorative, reconditioning, and rehabilitative services at medical treatment facilities in the United States. Nurses in this setting may participate in 20 or more surgeries per patient before the care is complete. Caring for the war wounded in any one of these settings involves continuous exposure to polytraumatic injuries, a multitude of environmental concerns, and complex organizational systems issues, each adding unique stressors to an already complex and dynamic clinical setting.

Ethics

To add to the complexity of the situation, morally distressing experiences may develop for the caregivers from the extreme conditions incurred during mass casualty conditions. Various situations encountered by nurses in all three echelons of care have raised questions about ethics and values. Some perioperative staff may feel conflicted about providing care to enemies and insurgents who have killed Americans. Some perioperative staff may feel conflicted about the quality of life left for survivors with extreme polytraumatic injuries. Providing perioperative nursing care to patients from a different culture with different values can be emotionally draining. Lack of supplies, danger, and discomfort can change how nurses view their work or their effectiveness in that work. Struggling with such issues adds another element of stress and may result in some type of grief response.

Some of the activated reserve staff have expressed frustration that, after being called up to help fight the global war on terrorism, they ended up working in surgery with warriors' family members and retirees. They have stated that they want to perform surgeries exclusively for the warriors, and no one else. These same individuals can be at risk for additional stress by not caring for the peacetime surgeries. When working on peace and war surgeries, a balance can be struck between the two so that the perioperative staff can

Box 1. Deployed stressors

Physical separation from family and friends for extended periods of time

Crossing time zones and feeling jet-lagged

Working in dangerous and filthy environments

Austere living conditions with lack of conveniences and privacy

Traveling under dangerous conditions

Never feeling "really safe" when working or resting

Inability to sleep with temperatures reaching 130°F (often resulting in fatigue)

Extremely cold temperatures leading to lethargy and the need for excessive sleep

Sandstorms and other unpleasant environmental conditions

Threats of chemical, biologic, radiologic, and nuclear warfare

High rates of casualties for extended periods of time

Repeated exposure to fresh mutilating wounds with massive bleeding

Exposure to severe burns, partial amputations, and surreal head and facial injuries

Working to save life, limb, and eyesight first and foremost

Large number of casualties simultaneously (referred to in the military as mass casualty)

Unpredictable mass casualty situations with no other hospitals to refer to or staff to borrow

Intensive manpower requirements and coordination when arranging patient movement to Germany through the aeromedical evacuation system

Poor water quality, when large quantities of water are required for cleaning and sterilizing

Equipment incompatibility (working with 110 and 220 power sources)

Surgical supply shortages with no available substitutions or areas to borrow from

Working with limited hygiene items and facilities

Field sanitation issues with regard to food waste, human waste, and amputated body parts

Need to make quick ethical and moral decisions

Issues of trust with colleagues and leaders when disclosing personal and professional information and concerns

Treating all patients, including enemy forces and insurgents, with the same standard of care

Treating host-nation people the best way possible, knowing that their country's infrastructure has little to help them in any rehabilitative recovery efforts; limited chance of another country assuming responsibility for the care

Team members entering and leaving the mission at different times

Feeling a lack of control over many of the workplace conditions

experience a healthy balance and develop their own resiliency to the stressors they encounter. Another consideration for the mental health of the perioperative staff is who they can go to when needing to express these feelings. If they were deployed with a large group of people they were accustomed to working with on their drill weekends, they may have a strong bond with several other staff members in a similar situation. If they were deployed alone or with a small team, they may not have many staff readily available to understand their point of view. The same can be true once they redeploy and return home to their civilian jobs. Who is there for them to talk to? Who is there who would understand what they were talking about?

Those reserve perioperative nurses and technicians called to be on active duty with the military who came from trauma centers in their civilian jobs have commented that, although they were accustomed to working with trauma surgeries in larger American cities, it was with a different population, and with a different set of circumstances. These perioperative nurses have shared that, although they thought they knew what to expect with war trauma, they actually were not prepared for the polytrauma on healthy athletic adults who trained professionally to be placed in those dangerous environments. The nurses were used to more irresponsible, preventable, gang, and

Box 2. Forward stressors

Separation from family and friends (for some staff members)

Repeated exposure to human tragedy, suffering, and polytrauma of younger people who suddenly have to live with life-altering challenges

Repeated exposure to mutilation injuries, burns, irrigation, wash-outs, and organ harvesting

Moving patients through the hospital back to the United States within 48 to 72 hours of receiving them from down-range (lack of closure in regard to the rest of the story)

Balancing numerous peacetime surgeries that may have an extended backlog time because of processing and performing war-related surgeries first

Sorting through European standards and American standards with regard to vendor manufacturer written instructions for products

Communicating with professional organizations or vendors with time zone differences

Greater dependence on ordering and processing loaner instrument sets from various vendors

Setting new policies for ordering an unpredictable number and unfamiliar style of implantable surgical devices

Deciding what purchasing agreements are best for supplying an increased demand for services and durable items

Being held to host-nation rules regarding sterilants and recycling laws

High staff and leadership turnover and turbulence

Working with multiple military services with different scopes of practice for their technical staff

Working with an ever-changing team with various expectations and work habits

Short-term assignment of surgical team members for 3 to 9 months who require time-intensive orientation, training, and personnel actions

New leadership, often creating a new vision and mission statement, and changing workplace expectations and priorities in the middle of the staff's tour of duty

Need to make quick ethical and moral decisions

Issues of trust with colleagues and leaders when disclosing personal and professional information and concerns

No opportunity to break or regroup by closing the operating room down

hoodlum behaviors and environments, and were used to dealing with trauma, but not multiple system traumas such as war can bring. Several nurses have commented that they did not expect to see such multiple and complex trauma surgeries concurrently happening at such a rate. These perioperative nurses spoke of the stressors and strains of watching the war wounded arrive in what seemed to be endless busloads, hearing their stories, all the while reminding them of their own children, friends, or relatives. The perioperative nurses and technicians spoke about being exposed to human tragedy at a level and for a time period they did not expect to encounter. They did not expect to be seeing on a daily basis the wounds caused by vehicle roll-overs, combined with burns, combined with gunshot wounds, combined with blast injuries, combined with traumatic amputations, combined with deglovings, combined with eye enucleations and other facial deformities, combined with multiple fragment injuries, combined with peppering injuries, combined with potential organ harvests. These multiple traumatic injuries were not caused by young people over-indulging in some type of joyride, but were happening to young athletic warriors trained in the art of war. These types of value judgments reflect societal values, and should be acknowledged and talked about.

The war environment can also bring with it a different process for triaging patients than is performed at civilian trauma centers. Depending on the location of the hospital, the resources, specialty expertise, and number and variety of other patients will enter into the equation quite differently. The hospital leadership will be faced with difficult decisions, and the staff need to be prepared to carry out those decisions to the best of their ability. At war, all patients, regardless of

---

Box 3. Stateside stressors

Repeated exposure to human tragedy, suffering, and polytrauma of younger people who suddenly have to live with life-altering challenges

Repeated exposure to mutilation injuries, burns, and progressive "whittling"

Performing surgery up to 20 times or more on the same patient

Undergoing public scrutiny and major publicity that may not tell the whole story about the institution and its work

Feeling that you are not really part of the war effort

Long, intensive, and demanding hours that often cut into family and personal time

Trying to balance the war and peace surgery schedules so all beneficiaries receive the best care possible

Greater dependence on ordering and processing loaner instrument sets from various vendors

Trained and experienced military members deploying on short notice, resulting in staffing shortages because back-fill staff do not arrive immediately

High staff and leadership turnover and turbulence

Working with an ever-changing team with various expectations and work habits

Short-term assignment of surgical team members for 3 to 9 months who require time-intensive orientation, training, and personnel actions

New leadership, often creating a new vision and mission statement, and changing workplace expectations and priorities in the middle of the staff's tour of duty

Feeling anxious and worried about the health, safety, and welfare of deployed colleagues and friends

Feeling guilty about being safe at home while friends and colleagues are deployed (and potentially in danger)

Need to make quick ethical and moral decisions

Issues of trust with colleagues and leaders when disclosing personal and professional information and concerns

Not receiving the same type of accolades, recognition, and appreciation as the deployed and forward workgroups

No opportunity to break or regroup by closing the operating room down

---

which country they are from, or whose side they are on are treated and triaged to the same standard of care. That always sounds wonderful until the last ventilator has been used, or the last wound vacuum-assisted closure device has been placed in a patient (Boxes 1–3).

Two main strategies help military perioperative nurses in coping with the enormous demands, challenges, and stressors encountered in the contemporary environment. A significant aspect of these two strategies is that they are interdependent. The features of one support and enhance the potential for success in the other. The first is the self-care plan and the second is the organizational care plan [6].

A self-care plan is a helpful and productive approach for nurses in dealing with their intense and ongoing stressors. The self-care plan is developed by using the basic foundation of a healthy diet, regular exercise, and proper sleep. From that point, each individual builds on his or her strengths and takes full advantage of all available resources and support systems [6].

Equally as important as the self-care plan is the organizational care plan that integrates the concepts of group morale, cohesion, teamwork, and pride. Internal support in an organization speaks volumes by recognizing its members as valuable and important. Structured support programs in the workplace help individuals and groups adapt in the face of adversity. Such programs have a high potential of affecting the health and fitness of the staff positively, increasing job satisfaction, improving retention, and enhancing the overall mission accomplishment through organizational effectiveness and productivity [6].

Tables 1 to 7 [4–12] outline (1) the various settings for military perioperative nurses, as previously defined in this article; (2) situations, conditions, or experiences; and (3) techniques and strategies for effective coping (on the far right side). Suggested recommendations in the far right

Table 1
Coping in the polytrauma clinical environment

Setting	Situation, condition, or experience	Techniques and strategies for individual and organizational care plans
Deployed Forward Stateside	Exposure to demanding, challenging, and stressful conditions often involving human trauma, injury, and illness Ongoing environmental, physical, and interpersonal stressors Ongoing systems-related issues and problems	Identify the importance and value of stress management, positive coping, and healthy adaptation [7,8] Identify all internal and external support systems and resources [6] Develop your individual care plan using creativity and innovation; implement your self care plan; revise as needed Build your resilience, defined by Birk [9] as raising tolerance so that stressful situations have less impact on the body and mind Strive to increase your inner strength and confidence Develop and sustain the ability to persevere during complex times and hardships [10] Develop and initiate an organizational care plan with your nursing colleagues; implement the organizational care plan with a focus on team building, cohesion, group morale, and positive interpersonal relationships in the workplace; revise as needed

column include individual actions and organizational measures.

At this point, it is recognized that stressors need to be identified, whether they are interpersonal, environmental, physical, or otherwise. These stressors have been identified in both wartime and natural disaster time situations. Stress indexes in the literature will give a score once the individual numbers are totaled, and that is the type of model that is being constructed to measure staff resiliency. We are working today in the living laboratories of what it means to build staff resiliency. At what point should a manager worry about staff when told that they are unable to eat or sleep the way they were used to, and that they no longer want to wake up and go to work? How does the manager separate out the true story of stressors from the potential malingerers and drama queens?

One protective and enhancing factor that can be put into place immediately is to foster positive interpersonal dynamics and respect within the work group. Positive experiences and relationships help in mission accomplishment. Treating the staff with compassion and kindness is the first step. Working in collaboration versus opposition allows the staff to capitalize on each others' strengths.

Staff resiliency programs are new to the military, and the information could easily transfer to the staff who respond to natural disaster situations. The Walter Reed Army Institute of Research wrote that people seek and thrive on validation and sincere appreciation. (Battlemind). The preliminary feedback from participants is positive.

Combat operational stress response and staff resiliency

Commonly reported thoughts, feelings, and behaviors from perioperative nurses and technicians working in military facilities at all echelons have included the following: difficulty concentrating, always feeling tired even when getting enough sleep, getting angry or easily irritated, feeling overwhelmed, increased cynicism, feeling discouraged, losing a sense of humor, not wanting to go to work (Elizabeth A.P. Vane, LTC, AN, RN, MS, CNOR and Mary S. Hull, LTC, AN, RN, MS, PMH-NP, personal communication, 2003–2007).

"Resiliency allows you to recover quickly from change, hardship, or misfortune. Resilient people demonstrate flexibility, durability, an attitude of optimism, and openness to learning. A lack of

Table 2
Elements of effective leadership

Setting	Situation, condition, or experience	Techniques and strategies for individual and organizational care plans
Deployed Forward Stateside	Perceptions of limited support from leaders	Organizational care plan (leader actions) Provide effective communication, including upward, downward, and lateral information [11] Make expectations clear [5] Plan carefully and thoroughly Be decisive and assertive Commit the group members to work that is commensurate with their training and experience Demonstrate effective leadership to earn the confidence, loyalty, and trust of subordinates [11] Encourage members to identify meaning and purpose in relation to their service Let every member know that he/she is valued and appreciated Initiate and support stress management programs [7] Promote functional, healthy, and supportive relationships among peers (commonly referred to as a battle buddy in the army, a wing man in the air force, and a shipmate in the navy) Foster a climate that encourages seeking help for problems [11] Encourage staff members to maintain contact with consultants and professional nursing organizations when practice questions arise or advice is needed Participate in specialized leader education and training in topics related to psychologic health and supportive strategies [7]

resilience is signaled by burnout, fatigue, malaise, depression, defensiveness, and cynicism" [10].

Civilian and military nurses are most likely to leave their jobs because of dissatisfaction with their front-line supervisor or because of work-related issues [13–15]. A practice environment that fosters communication, empowerment, and shared problem solving improves morale and increases retention and growth [16–19].

At one of the army medical centers, the concept of having a combat operational stress reaction/staff resiliency (COSR/SR) team has been successful since 2006. The team is composed of chaplains, behavioral health staff, nursing staff, and social workers who voluntarily reach out to hospital personnel. For instance, the operating room and sterile processing department staff have the names and contact information of the

Table 3
Awareness of situational and workplace danger

Setting	Situation, condition, or experience	Techniques and strategies for individual and organizational care plans
Deployed	Threat of dangerous exposure	Organizational care plan Create a binding force (group cohesion) that keeps group members together in performing the mission despite the possibility of danger [11] Develop and supervise safety policies and procedures [5] Institute all possible protective measures [5] Conduct rugged and realistic training [11] Focus on adaptation through readiness; readiness as defined by Reineck [4] (p.253) is "a dynamic concept with dimensions at the individual, group, and system levels, which, together, influence one's ability to prepare to accomplish the mission"

Table 4
Group cohesiveness

Setting	Situation, condition, or experience	Techniques and strategies for individual and organizational care plans
Deployed Forward Stateside	Potential to become physically, emotionally, or spiritually fatigued	**Individual care plan** Maintain physical exercise, a healthy diet, proper hydration, and adequate sleep Leisure activities and hobbies (which are limited in the deployed setting, thus requiring extreme creativity and innovation) Maintain a sense of humor Build on your strengths Maintain healthy relationships; spend time with people who give you positive energy [10] If separated from family because of mobilization or deployment, remain in contact by e-mail, phone calls, letter writing Use your spiritual beliefs or faith-based system when struggling or coping with difficulty
Deployed	Potential to become physically, emotionally, or spiritually fatigued	**Organizational care plan** Recognize that deployed nurses not only work together but live together during continuous operations, thus creating extremely stressful conditions Remember that all members are separated from their primary support systems and might need assistance from time to time Develop a unit sleep-management program that allows soldiers at least 6 hours, and preferably 7 to 8, for sleep out of every 24; sleep does not need to be continuous but uninterrupted sleep is preferred [11]. Organize group leisure activities (such as movies, card games, board games); group sporting events (such as volleyball); arts and crafts Recognize special events and achievements; celebrate holidays and birthdays; Encourage journal clubs and book clubs Undertake other creative and innovative team-building activities designed by the group to maintain group integrity and connectivity Use all mental health assets in the area of operations (psychology nurses and technicians, social workers, psychologists, psychiatrists, and occupational therapists) for building psychologic fitness and resilience [7] Invite chaplains and ministry teams to participate actively in the organizational care plan and to be available for staff; be mindful that a chaplain's assistant is needed for the chaplain's protection because chaplains do not carry weapons (ie, two bodies are needed wherever a chaplain is needed)
Forward Stateside	Potential to become physically, emotionally, or spiritually fatigued	**Organizational care plan** Recognize special events and achievements; hold holiday staff parties Encourage journal clubs Organize team-building activities during staff meetings or as part of continuing education and professional development activities Use all mental health assets in the area of operations (psychology nurses and technicians, social workers, psychologists, psychiatrists, and occupational therapists) for building psychologic fitness and resilience [7] Invite chaplains and ministry teams to participate actively in the organizational care plan and to be available for staff

Table 5
Stress recognition to enhance coping

Setting	Situation, condition, or experience	Techniques and strategies for individual and organizational care plans
Deployed Forward Stateside	Potential for ineffective and maladaptive coping; potential for stress responses	Individual care plan It is extremely important to recognize and accept all feelings, including uncomfortable ones [10] Anger, anxiety, sadness, and grief are natural and expected during the lived experience; addressing such feelings in a constructive, productive, and goal-oriented fashion can be accomplished through discussion with a trusted individual (friend, family member, colleague, mental health provider, or clergy) Embrace the situation with courage, compassion, and confidence A simple, but powerful technique for self care is journal writing; journaling helps the writer manage feelings and provides a medium for self reflection; journaling promotes awareness and cultivates insight and wisdom [10,12] Identify the meaning, purpose, and value of your work; nurses who derive positive feelings from their experiences are able to demonstrate effective coping and adaptation [10] Respond to stressful situations based on your core beliefs and value system; view stressful experiences as growth opportunities [9] Respond to stressful situations based on the values of the organization; for the military these include Army values: loyalty, duty, respect, selfless service, honor, integrity, personal courage Air force values: integrity first, service before self, excellence in all we do Navy values: honor, courage, commitment
Deployed Forward Stateside	Potential for ineffective and maladaptive coping; potential for stress responses	Organizational care plan Focus on methods for developing strong personal trust, loyalty, and cohesiveness between peers and coworkers (horizontal bonding) [11] Focus on methods for developing strong personal trust, loyalty, and cohesiveness between leaders and subordinates (vertical bonding) [11] Understand the importance of the above-stated relationships and how they contribute to organizational success

Table 6
Need for continuous team building

Setting	Situation, condition, or experience	Techniques and strategies for individual and organizational care plans
Deployed Forward Stateside	Rapid turnover of personnel	Organizational care plan Ensure new arrivals are welcomed into the unit, helping them to become known and trusted Assign a sponsor to the new group member Encourage experienced members to teach, coach, and mentor Ensure new member understands his/her job and is properly trained Allow adequate overlap time between the incoming and outgoing staff

Table 7
Conflict resolution for team building

Setting	Situation, condition, or experience	Techniques and strategies for individual and organizational care plans
Deployed Forward Stateside	Interpersonal conflict in the workplace	Organizational care plan Recognize that interpersonal conflict is inevitable and will arise to some degree in the workplace Focus on conflict resolution techniques such as assertiveness, open and honest communication, seeking to understand the other person's point of view Remain nonjudgmental; treat others with dignity and respect; remain solution focused

chaplains and social workers assigned to their areas posted in their break rooms for ready access. The overarching goal of this team is to provide assistance to the staff for coping and adaptation so the staff can become more resilient. Raising an individual's tolerance so that stressful situations have less impact on the body and mind is called building resilience [9]. Resiliency gives the staff the ability to persevere during difficult times and during hardships. Resiliency increases the inner strength and confidence of the staff.

Combat operational stress reactions are best described as the expected and predictable intellectual, emotional, physical, and behavioral reactions from exposure to difficult, challenging, and demanding conditions [11]. These reactions can happen in the wartime environment, or during times of natural disasters, while providing patient care with the enormous demands and challenges that are faced daily.

The COSR team is able to give advice on how to deal with irritability, trouble falling asleep or remaining asleep, grief, anxiety, and fatigue. These consultations are done without the staff having their careers placed in jeopardy or having their concerns made public. Should additional measures be needed, all efforts are placed on staff anonymity. The COSR team will try every available preventive measure, supportive discussion, or educational tool, and will offer extensive guidance to move that individual staff member in the right direction.

The COSR team is also equipped to organize and run larger discussion groups, brown bag lunches, workshops, presentations, team-building activities, and consultation with the leadership to build a supportive work environment. They are also able to work with the "drive-by hallway" consultations.

The COSR team meets weekly to talk about common trends they are seeing within the organization and the concerns of individuals and work groups. Working together, they are able to use a preventive, proactive, and constructive approach to meet the needs of the staff.

In conclusion, mental fitness is equally as important as the technical and tactical proficiency, physical fitness, physical health, and operational knowledge required for polytrauma wartime surgeries, or those in times of natural disaster. Building staff resiliency is paramount to building and retaining competent and qualified staff. The issues the authors present in this article are real. The staff and their stories are real, with real families, real homes to maintain, and real support systems that they use to deal with multiple stressors. Training and educating perioperative nurse managers to be alert to signs of fatigue and other stressors, to be flexible with work patterns and ideas while upholding national standards, and to be available and able to work with all staff in problem solving can lead to better team building and greater resiliency, which ultimately leads to better patient care. Caring for the caregiver is essential in the global war on terrorism and during natural disasters; these situations create similar stressors and demands on the perioperative nursing staff.

References

[1] AORN. Standards, recommended practices, and guidelines, with official AORN statements. Denver (CO): Association of periOperative Registered Nurses; 2007. p. 16, 83, 398, 399.
[2] Gaba DM, Howard SK. Patient safety; fatigue among clinicians and the safety of patients. N Engl J Med 2002;347(16):1249–55.

[3] Rosekind MR, Gander PH, Gregory KB, et al. Managing fatigue in operational setting 1: physiological considerations and counter-measures. Hosp Top 1997;75(3):23–30.

[4] Reineck C. Individual readiness in nursing. Mil Med 1999;164(4):251–5.

[5] Vane E, Drost E, Elder D, et al. Behind the scenes: patient safety in the operating room and central materiel service during deployments. Advances in Patient Safety from research to implementation 2005. vol 3, Implementation issues. 469–82.

[6] Kenny D, Hull M. Critical care nurses' experience in caring for the casualties of war evacuated from the front line lessons learned and needs identified. Crit Care Nurs Clin North Am; in press.

[7] The Department of Defense plan to achieve the vision of the Department of Defense Task Force on Mental Health, report to congress. September 2007.

[8] Department of the Army Landstuhl Regional Medical Center Division of Behavioral Health, Memorandum for Chief, United States Army Nurse Corp, Office of the Surgeon General, Subject: Proposal for the creation of a staff advocacy Officer position. 25 June 2007.

[9] Birk M. Resilient people learn to bounce back from stress. Mercury 2007;34(7).

[10] Pulley ML, Wakefield M. For the practicing manager, building resiliency, how to thrive in times of change. Greensboro (NC): Center for Creative Leadership; 2001.

[11] Department of the Army (DA). Combat and operational stress control. Washington (DC): Headquearters Department of the Army; 2006; Field Manual 4–02.51.

[12] Mulligan L. Overcoming compassion fatigue. Kans Nurse 2004;79(7) [Journal Chapter, Pictorial].

[13] Force M. The relationship between effective nurse managers and nursing retention. J Nurs Adm 2005; 35(7–8):336–41.

[14] McGuire E, Kennerly S. Nurse managers as transformational and transactional leaders. Nurs Econ 2006;24(4):179–85.

[15] Upenieks V. What constitutes effective leadership? Perceptions of magnet and nonmagnet nurse leaders. J Nurs Adm 2003;33(9):456–67.

[16] Kerfoot K. Reliability between nurse managers: the key to the high-reliability organization. Nurs Econ 2006;24(5):274–5.

[17] Stedman M, Nolan T. Coaching: a different approach to the nursing dilemma. J Nurs Adm 2007;31(1):43–9.

[18] Thomka L. Mentoring and its impact on intellectual capital: through the eyes of the mentee. J Nurs Adm 2007;31(1):22–6.

[19] Wagner S. Staff retention: from "satisfied" to "engaged". Nurs Manage 2006;37(3):24–9.

ELSEVIER
SAUNDERS

Perioperative Nursing Clinics 3 (2008) 85–90

PERIOPERATIVE
NURSING
CLINICS

Musings on Health Care Design Research for Surgery

A. Ray Pentecost III, DrPH, AIA, ACHA*

Clarx Nexsen, 6160 Kempsville Circle, Suite 200-A, Norfolk, VA 23502, USA

Within the lifetimes of many surgical teams practicing today, surgical interventions will dramatically decrease and be increasingly limited to the domains of obstetrics, trauma and elective plastics, and organ and joint replacements. Except for trauma cases, unanticipated surgeries will virtually disappear because of the accurate predictive modeling of health care demand resulting from genome decoding and full-body diagnostic and reference imaging. Digital three-dimensional virtual exploratory procedures from multiple modalities yielding scalable and manipulable images will be fully integrated with noninvasive interventional technologies. Waves and beams will render obsolete many traditional invasive exploratory–interventional models of care. Surgeries will increasingly be robot-assisted because of economic forces to reduce costs and the pressure to reduce the number of medication and procedural errors. Because of the reduction in the number of procedures and concern about infection-related mortality rates in health care facilities, surgeries will be conducted in sterile, not just a clean, environments. Workers will celebrate the safer workplaces that boast fewer incidents of injury and disease among surgical staff.

As surgery undergoes this technology-driven sea-change in practice, the design of health care architecture is also undergoing enormous transformation, moving quickly and enthusiastically from the "I've always done it that way" and "We have every reason to believe this" period of thoughtful, but relatively imprecise, design into the "Where is the research to prove that position" era. Architects call it evidence-based design (EBD)

after the parallel mindset in medicine that takes its identity from the initiative to build best medical practices out of evidentiary findings, not anecdotal sensibilities. The central theme of the EBD movement is the belief that research into the impact that the built environment has on the healing process can actually provide information on how to build environments that improve or enhance the healing experience for patients, staff, and family. It has already had a significant impact on the practice of health care architecture.

The great challenge to medical architecture researchers is how to set an EBD research agenda in the midst of this dramatic and fast-moving change. Although abandoning short-term research to focus on the enormous and tantalizing changes looming on the horizon is tempting, visionary posturing is never ultimately satisfying to researchers because it studies a reality that never really arrives. The future is always just beyond reach. Instead, it is in researching improvements to current practice while at the same time effectively laying the foundation for the future that the art of "asking the right question" emerges.

In this swirling context of overwhelming change to both the surgical and medical architectural professions, the invitation to write about some of the major research frontiers in surgical design is at first overwhelming. The notion of a design professional writing to a readership of highly trained medical specialists who know the operating room (OR) better than I ever will is a bit daunting, but while I am an architect I am not without portfolio in the OR. My career began in the OR as a surgical orderly while I was still in college studying architecture. My theory was simple: if one is going to design health care facilities, what better way to understand them than to work in them. This was my earliest

* Corresponding author.
  E-mail address: rpentecost@clarknexsen.com

1556-7931/08/$ - see front matter © 2008 Elsevier Inc. All rights reserved.
doi:10.1016/j.cpen.2007.11.010

journey into the world of health care design research.

It was a wonderful education, in many ways. For example, I discovered from one of the other orderlies that the architect must always prove himself to the client. He asked me what the silver strip running across the floor of the orderly dressing area was, and I will never forget the look he gave me when I correctly told him it was an expansion joint. He seemed almost disappointed that he did not stump me, but the hint of a smile immediately thereafter made it clear that I had made the grade and I could belong to the OR family. Now, as the Director of Health Care Architecture for a major architecture and engineering firm, I find that nothing has changed.

Operating room design

Consider the issues that will seriously impact surgical practice in the near future. First, medical technology futurists tell us that within our lifetimes the medical profession will evolve into something that resembles the financial industry. We will understand the influence of genetics and predisposition to disease so fully that patients will get a baseline genetic scan of some kind to take to a medical care advisor, who may or may not be a physician. From that will come a regimen of nutrition, exercise, and other kinds of recommendations aimed at keeping us healthy and steering us away from those things to which we are predisposed. In essence, absent the unfortunate and unpredictable traumatic event that requires immediate surgical intervention or lays the groundwork for a future need, individuals will have a strong sense of the kinds of medical procedures they can expect during our lifetimes.

When we can take a cohort of the population and predict with some clarity what their reasonable surgical demands are going to be in their lifetimes, both in terms of volume and types of procedures, planning for ORs will change. Also, it may also be that the number of ORs in a given health care system reflects less the ability to accommodate surprise surgical demand and more the predictable demand of those living in proximity of that facility or those enrolled in that facility's health plan.

People seem determined to experience accidents and have traumatic events in their lives that require surgical remedy. They have pregnancies that routinely present difficult delivery options made easier with surgery. Repair and enhancement procedures that overcome deficiencies in hearing, sight, orthopedic function, and heart arrhythmias, and that afford reconstruction after trauma or birth defect are being considered for the foreseeable future. But the question is how much of what is now considered inescapable demand for surgical procedures will be avoidable in the future?

Perhaps one of the most obvious illustrations for this issue is the treatment of cancer. Bioengineered remedies for cancer threaten to obviate the need for surgical intervention. Designed substances that constrain the growth of cancers, cut off the food supply to cancers and cause them to wither and die, and bind the cancer's ability to metastasize, all are nonsurgical interventions that are well into development and clinical trial. To what extent will today's medical research render the OR unnecessary because of the discovery of highly effective nonsurgical treatment options?

Short-term research issue

How can ORs be designed for effective and efficient changes in their traditional or initial use? One possibility is *universal design*, which refers to the notion that if you design an OR for the ultimate case, in terms of factors such as complexity, staffing, technological support, and special lighting, then it would theoretically be able to accommodate every kind of procedure, and the expectation is that the efficiency of an OR department increases. In practical terms, this rarely refers to a single OR design replicated en masse to form a surgical suite, but more often to a few standardized OR rooms able to accommodate clusters or families of procedures that are then reproduced to form a surgical suite. Research on the administrative and business implications of accommodating evolving surgical demand using a universal design model would be useful in making or breaking the argument in favor of this flexible design model.

Long-term research issue

How convertible are today's ORs, including any that might be universally designed, in light of reasonably anticipated obsolescence? This question invites study on structural grid and its ability to accommodate alternate hospital interiors, the reuse of the hospital infrastructure that accompanies an OR, and the challenge of downsizing the surgical suite without completely eliminating it.

Strategic and tactical studies on implementing a sea change in thinking in surgical practice would be valuable, particularly if it could begin to examine regional models of surgical demand that made regional conversions of surgical infrastructures a possibility versus facility-based conversions that might necessarily be less efficient and more costly.

Imaging in the operating room environment

Second, consider the increasing and absolutely vital role imaging has in all that is done in health care. It is already moving from an interesting and critically important component of traditional medical and surgical practice to a place of centrality in a digital patient information system around which all other patient information is oriented. Every patient procedure, test, trauma, reading, and inference is being linked to a body geocode, much like urban planning and development information is geocoded to a map, except that this will occur with a three-dimensional image of the body. Virtual exploratory technologies are already rendering unnecessary any kind of invasive approach to discovery.

Short-term research issue

In the OR, where imaging is already a dramatically expanding aspect of any surgical procedure, how are environments created that move imaging from its current assistive role in traditional surgeries into a more central role that renders traditional surgery unnecessary? Will those environments require the same attention to cleanliness and sterility that invasive rooms require? How extensive will a virtual surgical practice be in a typical general hospital? Will different staff requirements be needed? Will staff need to scrub the same way they do now? If a wave of non-invasive imaging diagnostics is emerging, how vulnerable is the hospital to an outmigration of those procedures to the physician's office?

Long-term research issue

Because imaging technologies are increasingly being integrated into noninvasive treatment modalities that use the same or related technologies as those that create the images, how can demand be accurately anticipated and where will the line need to be drawn between the imaging and surgical suites? Although imaging is closely related today to the surgical suite, and is occasionally interventional, it is increasingly going to be more than integral to the surgery; it will displace the surgery. Highly targetable technologies that minimize collateral damage to otherwise healthy tissue, allow a tighter and cleaner impact zone for the beam, and are virtually the same technologies as those that create the images of the pathologies will increasingly displace the need for traditional OR theaters.

Robotic technology

Third, the practical limits of robotics in surgery also must be understood. Where is the point at which the machine exceeds the ability of the human to keep up? The designers of jet fighters have lamented that in recent generations of fighters, the challenge is to manage the onboard computers to the point where the fighter pilots are able to keep up with the information processing requirements. Fighter pilots are arguably among the most capable multitaskers in any profession, but apparently even they have practical limits.

What about surgeons and their practical limits? I recently saw a video of a "robotic juke box circulating nurse" being used in a surgery. The robot simply went to the device that held various tools appropriate for that kind of surgery and removed whatever tool the surgeon requested. The challenge, according to the speaker, was managing the rest of the surgical experience so that the robot–human interface was successful. In fact, as we watched the video of the robot at work, the speaker disclosed that the video had been slowed down just to allow us to see clearly the movements of the robot, because at actual speed the movements might be blurred.

Short-term research issue

In keeping with the robotics theme, what are the practical limits of surgeon multiplication? It is not new to manage surgeries with highly trained teams that do some part of the surgery in preparation for the lead surgeon, who performs the specialized portion of the surgery, with the team closing that case while the lead surgeon moves on to the next. And robotics? How effectively can robotic technologies such as the da Vinci Surgical System (Intuitive Surgical, Inc., Sunnyvale, California), be used to multiply surgical resources at same-site and remote-site procedures? Architecturally, administratively, and medically, what is required to make these technologies effective vehicles for multiplying surgical capabilities? To what extent are these approaches limited by facilities, technologies, or personnel? Do these procedures require a hospital context for maximum safety and efficacy?

Long-term research issue

What is the role of this high-priced minimally invasive surgery (MIS) technology in the impending significantly reduced universe of surgical procedures? Will minimally invasive procedures always have a place or will they be largely displaced by molecular-scaled interventions? Will the environments that accommodate these technologies be reusable for something else? Will surgical robotics become a technology that is so specialized and facing such reduced demand that it survives only in regional centers? If so, what is the medical context that surrounds that technology in a supportive, noncompetitive dynamic: a hospital or physician's office or some hybrid health care facility that only caters to certain kinds of MIS procedures?

Operating room errors

Fourth, concern is growing about the errors that occur in health care facilities in general and surgery in particular. As a metric that is watched closely by safety officers in hospitals, it is an issue that begs study by those seeking ways to reduce medication and procedural errors in the OR. Much is being learned about medication error and, by extension, other kinds of seemingly simple mistakes made by health care workers. For example, it seems that better lighting can help staff in the management of medication errors, and a quieter environment with fewer distractions can also be helpful in reducing medication errors. Because these errors are costly, in terms of human capital and medical resources, the health care industry is keenly interested in environments that reduce error rates of all kinds, including those in surgery.

Short-term research issue

Studies must be conducted in surgery to explore ways to reduce errors of all kinds through environmental modifications, such as lighting, noise management, and the elimination of distractions wherever possible. Additionally, studying the technologic components of injury that the built environment will not overcome would be interesting. In other words, do some forces impact error rates that are not necessarily linked directly to the facility? For example, a medical model that leaves workers overworked and stressed can contribute to errors in the OR regardless of, or maybe despite, design features intended to remedy environmental influences that may contribute to errors.

Long-term research issue

To what extent will a reduced surgical load in the future reduce the opportunities for error in the OR? For example, will surgeries be anticipated to the extent that certain preparations can be made in advance or even off-site and brought to the OR with fewer errors? Will surgical facilities in the future be, to a greater degree, outside the traditional hospital and therefore in a less-distracting environment? To what extent will robotics contribute to a reduction in errors in the OR from less human-to-human interaction? To what degree can certain components of the surgical experience be moved elsewhere in the hospital and thereby subjected to fewer of the distractions of the OR?

Sterile environment

Fifth, what is the value of having a sterile environment in health care? For decades the push has been to make surgery a place of cleanliness: with the caps, gloves, shoe covers, the exhaustive scrubbing of the surgeon's hands, and the Betadine washes on surgical sites; the emphasis on purity is inescapable. But in what context does this focus on cleanliness exist?

Consider the new equipment being introduced into the market by STERIS called VaproSure Room Sterilizer. This portable device can be rolled into a room and left on for a short time, after which the room is effectively sterile. I recently had the opportunity to discuss this technology with a physician who cynically reminded me that even after the room was cleaned, it was only sterile until a person entered.

Although this is true, it really is not the question. The issue is whether value exists in returning the OR, patient room, or laboratory cubicle, after serving a patient known to have methicillin-resistant *Staphylococcus aureus*, *Clostridium difficile*, or vancomycin-resistant *Enterococcus*, back to a zero culture level before the next patient arrives or the next worker enters for routine activity.

Short-term research issue

What is the value of a clean room as a periodic benchmark in the struggle against the so-called "superbugs"? What are the administrative protocols that define when, how often, and before and after which cases a room should be thoroughly cleaned? What is the cost–benefit of taking a room off-line long enough to clean it before restoring it to active service in terms of reducing incidence of costly hospital acquired infections? The impact on patient through-put, staffing levels, disability, and litigation costs could be significant.

Long-term research issue

Will the greater influence on reduced infection rates in hospitals occur through room sterilization technology or simple medical staff behaviors, such as hand washing? To what extent hand washing, or other staff practices, can reduce exposure risks to highly infectious agents compared with transmission risks is unclear, and better understanding of that distinction will be key in determining the cost–benefit findings on any of the new sterilization technologies. To what extent will sterile become the industry standard compared with simply very clean? How can facility designers create spaces that are easier to clean or easier to sterilize?

Safety

Sixth, I must also acknowledge my passion for creating safer health care workplaces. Injuries caused by avoidable causes still occur at an alarming rate. The design of a safer OR must continue to be a priority. Patient transfers in the OR are a serious matter impacting worker safety, and I have mentioned infection management technologies that affect not just patient but also worker safety. The issue of safety in the health care workplace even extends to the design of medical devices. The disposal of sharps, for example, demands creative research that goes beyond red collection boxes and retractable needles. Infection control cannot be as simple as periodic room sterilization; it must extend into routine medical behaviors protecting patients and workers. The number of bariatric patients is increasing with alarming statistics on how many citizens are now overweight. Moving these individuals, even slightly, can place workers at serious risk for injury.

One new technology that holds some promise for improving worker safety is the patient transport device that functions as a gurney and a surgical platform. Several manufacturers are introducing these technologies in hopes of minimizing back injuries in workers and exposure to falls by patients. To what degree this technology is actually impacting those injury risks is unclear.

Short-term research issue

Where is the greatest exposure to the risk for injury to workers in surgery, and is the answer to this risk a technology, a new behavior, a new design concept, or some combination of the three? Does the technology to reduce the exposure to injury exist or must it be invented? How does the staff model contribute to injuries in the OR where roles are fairly explicit and crossing over to help a coworker is not always the norm? How can the architecture contribute to and reinforce safer behaviors?

Long-term research issue

How will the nursing shortage influence the increasing use of technologies in surgery? Will more lifts be used to move patients when nurses are fewer and older? Will robotics do more of the heavy lifting of materials and patients, and will they enable hospitals to deploy longer OR schedules because the staff will not experience as much fatigue? Will the nursing shortage increase the cost of staff so much that hospital-acquired infection and other worker safety and health risks will drive medical practices to a higher, and more costly level of worker protection, and how will the design of ORs contribute to that safety?

Supportive work environments

And seventh, in closing, I would like to suggest that all workers associated with surgery would benefit from some serious research into what kinds of surgical environments are most supportive of workers in nonclinical terms. Given the shortage of nursing staff, their increasing mean age, and their clear expression of lifestyle as a priority, the entire medical community must think about how to handle them. If the costs of recruitment, overtime, contract labor, and temporary workers are factored into the cost of health care, including surgical care, then the importance of this issue, in monetary terms at least, becomes even clearer.

Short-term research issue

What types of ORs are the most pleasant places to work? What features in the OR contribute most to worker satisfaction? Is an OR with a view to the outside, or a floor that is soft and easier on the feet and spine, or various environmental controls for ambient light, music or white noise, temperature, or other environmental dimensions, such as color, the most comfortable? Is a quiet OR, or an OR with robots that have displaced staff in the more stressful job positions the most pleasant? How does OR design influence the cost of OR staffing?

Long-term research issue

Does any real correlation exist between surgical worker satisfaction and worker safety, or between worker satisfaction and worker recruiting and retention? All other research issues aside, this may rise to the level of urgency, because in an era of nursing staff shortages any studies that provide insights for how to improve nurse recruiting, retention, and satisfaction are of immediate interest and applicability. Prioritizing the clinical aspect of the workings of health care facilities at the expense of appropriate care and attention to the workers themselves is tempting, but may it never be said of the health care design community that the health care worker was ignored or diminished in priority to any other person in the health care equation.

Summary

The frontiers of blended medical and architectural research are rich. Worthy topics may outstrip the capability of the research community to pursue them, but EBD is a movement focused squarely on advancing research-driven health care design. The hunger for insights on the most effective ways to create healing environments will not soon diminish.

Acknowledgments

The author gratefully acknowledges the help of Peter L. Bardwell, FAIA, FACHA and Bruce Bonine, AIA, ACHA in the advance research for and, ultimately, in the preparation of this article.

ELSEVIER
SAUNDERS

Perioperative Nursing Clinics 3 (2008) 91–94

PERIOPERATIVE
NURSING
CLINICS

Ambient Nature Sounds in Health Care

Chip Davis, BA[a], George F. Nussbaum, PhD, RN, CNOR[b],*

[a]*Mannheim Steamroller, 9130 Mormon Bridge Road, Omaha, NE 68152, USA*
[b]*Graduate School of Nursing, Perioperative Clinical Nurse Specialist Program,
Uniformed Services University, 4301 Jones Bridge Road, Bethesda, MD 20814, USA*

The use of music and sound has been recognized throughout history as beneficial and therapeutic. The Ancient Romans and Greeks in Epidaurus believed music had the power to heal body, mind, and spirit. The shepherd David, from biblical times, calmed the mind of King Saul with his harp. In more recent times clinical studies have shown the efficiency of music therapy for perioperative patients from multiple cultures and age ranges [1]. Sound or music seems to stimulate involuntary centers in the central nervous system, causing a physiologic response that subsequently influences conscious thought. Music may be transmitted initially to higher levels of the brain where sound affects emotional and abstract thought before physiologic responses occur [1].

Recently published, randomized, controlled clinical studies show the potential of a therapeutic milieu that decreases anxiety and increases the threshold for pain in conscious patients. One study using intraoperative music provided by headphone to patients under general anesthesia found no change in surgical stress in terms of plasmatic levels of norepinephrine, epinephrine, cortisol, or adrenocorticotropic hormone [2]. Other studies using music and sound on conscious patients in the immediate pre- and postoperative periods indicate a positive effect in modulating the physiologic response to stress and pain [3–12].

Sense of place

The understanding that *place* has a significant influence on health is not new. Centuries ago,

Hippocrates, in *Airs, Waters, and Places*, taught his students to distinguish unhealthy places, such as swamps, from healthy places, such as sunny, breezy hillsides [13].

Today, the term *place* connotes its atmosphere and the quality of its environment. This entity is significant because "...we recognize that certain localities have an attraction which gives us a certain indefinable sense of well-being and which we want to return to, time and again. Places can evoke memories, arouse emotions, and excite passions" [13].

Psychoacoustics and ambient therapy

Psychoacoustics is the study of subjective perception of sounds in the environment. It explains the subjective response of the listener to the surrounding location and circumstances. It is the intermediary in acoustical concerns because an individual's response to sound is what is important. Psychoacoustics reconciles acoustical stimuli with the objective and physical properties that are associated with them and with the physiologic and psychological responses induced by them. Ambient sound technology applies the principles of psychoacoustics—the ability to create spatial perceptions through the interrelationships of sound, hearing, and the "mind's eye."

Ambient therapy combines specially recorded sounds of nature with distinctive music content that helps guide emotional perceptions. Actualized through sophisticated electronic technology and based on recording algorithms, the programs may be able to mentally transport patients from their hospital or clinical setting to a different, positive environment. Ambient therapy has the goal of counteracting feelings of anxiety and

* Corresponding author.
E-mail address: nussbaumgf@verizon.net
(G.F. Nussbaum).

1556-7931/08/$ - see front matter
doi:10.1016/j.cpen.2007.11.007

isolation, and other negative distractions through replacing them with an overall sense of comfort and well-being. *Ambient music therapy* refers to a combination of natural sounds recorded to create different, distracting audio spaces that mask the transient startle sounds of the hospital environment with the drone of natural environmental sounds. The principle of ambient music therapy is to have patient's imagine they are in the place they are hearing through having them get involved with the music, thereby putting their mind at ease through distraction.

Elements that contribute to this phenomenon of ambient music are noise floor, delay time shift/ space perception, and range of emotions. A certain amount of ambient noise is present every day, which is considered *noise floor*. Sounds that disrupt are referred to as *startle sounds*. These sounds are high transient spikes in the normal pattern of surrounding sounds, such as a door slam or gunshot. The drone of consistency can provide a sense of well-being. Therefore, if a drone of natural sounds can be created, they may mask the transient, startle sounds. This technique may be useful for treatments that require patients to be at ease for the greatest benefit (Fig. 1).

Examples of an ambient noise floor cover exists in many natural places. Ambient therapy uses natural sounds to create a psychoacoustic experience. Because people are products of nature, a sympathetic chord seems to ring within everyone when exposed to these types of sounds, making ambient therapy sounds more believable.

People hear in two different ways: the ears are "hardwired" to hear nature sounds and never shut off, creating an internal alarm system, whereas music is recognized in a more "executive function" of the brain.

Audio signals move faster through nerve fibers than pain signals. Because of the gating

mechanism in the nerve fibers, only a certain amount of information can flow at any given time. If a certain amount of signal space is taken up by the faster-moving audio signals, less gate room may be available for pain signals. People have a natural connection to nature sounds; they innately mean something to each individual. People have the natural ability to distinguish and recognize the intensity of sounds in forward and backward directions.

The technology used in creating ambient music therapy involves placing microphones in multiple nature-intense environments 200 ft apart and creating a time-delayed algorithm. Through creating this unique algorithm, a 20-ft × 20-ft hospital room recreates actual sounds as if the patient was lying in the forest, mountain stream, or ocean coastline. The idea is to create a less-confining space and add to the patient's sense of well-being, as shown in Fig. 2.

When patients believe they are in a certain place, their mood and psyche adjust and compensate for behavior related to their perception of this place. This phenomenon is what is meant by ambient therapy addressing the range of emotions. In music, certain patterns of notes can address different emotions, as shown in Fig. 3.

The purpose of psychoacoustics, using ambience, is for patients to begin believing they are in a different environment, such as in a sun-drenched spring forest as opposed to a hospital waiting room. When individuals begin believing they are

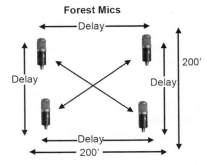

Fig. 2. Recording technique of ambient nature sounds. Using technologically sophisticated recording equipment, sounds in nature were captured to create ambient beds to minimize spikes or startle sounds. Musical elements have been added that spring from the nature sounds to address emotions. The microphones are placed 200 ft apart, so that in a 20-ft × 20-ft room the delay time/algorithm is 200 ft, just like being in a forest or other natural environment.

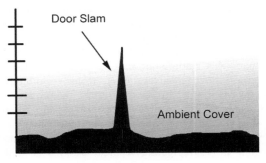

Fig. 1. Ambient noise floor.

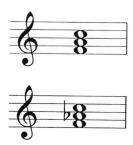

Fig. 3. Major and minor chords. Major chords tend to evoke happiness and well-being, whereas minor chords imply sadness.

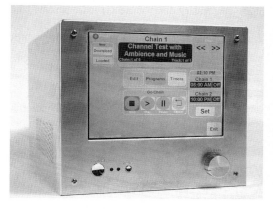

Fig. 4. Ambient therapy system. (*Courtesy of* Ambience Medical, Omaha, NE; with permission.)

in a certain place, their mood and psyche adjust to and compensates for behavior related to their perception of that place. When the psyche begins to believe what the acoustic surroundings suggest, emotions can be guided with music.

Ambient music therapy is not the same as other music therapy modalities, although music is involved. This type of music has the combination of natural sounds in combination with musical parts created to move the emotional parts of the whole person creating a sense of relaxation and well-being. The basic goal in health care is to put patients or others involved at ease through distraction. In physical therapy, the term *range of motion* is applied. In ambient therapy, nature sounds and music can be applied to address the range of emotion. If the ambient noise floor has become believable, an individual will begin believing they are where their ears tell them they are.

The ambient therapy delivery system

The Ambient Therapy System (ATS) was developed to deliver the ambient therapy algorithm in a clear and predictable way (Fig. 4). The ATS can play back the various seasonal natural algorithms and musical content, balance the room dimensions to place the patient in the proper listening position, and receive additional programming as it becomes available.

Ambient therapy combines specially recorded sounds of nature with distinctive music content to provide patients with a new perceptual reality, an environment designed to be soothing and comforting that perhaps can counteract feelings of pain, anxiety, and isolation. Unique to ambient therapy is its audio system: a portable console and accompanying surround sound system that applies the concepts of psychoacoustics.

Research opportunities

Current research with ambient therapy differs significantly from other studies using music therapy alone. Most of the studies cited previously used headphones to deliver the therapy to patients. Other studies allowed participants to select the specific musical genre they wished to hear. The ambient system, as the term implies, uses a unique system (ATS) to deliver the acoustical surround sound into the room rather than through headsets.

Clinical trials are being performed in a children's oncology center, in a spinal cord rehabilitation center, and with patients experiencing postoperative pain after coronary artery bypass. The hypothesis is that environments providing nature sounds and background music specific for the population being studies will reduce anxiety associated with the clinical condition, the pain intensity, and the requirement for pain medication. Previous studies cited in clinical trials and the current trials using ambient therapy have not adequately validated the research designs or methodologies for measuring the potential effect of music or the sound environment on patient response to therapy or the effect on nursing staff providing the care to these individuals. However, research-developed tools that test pain and anxiety are available, and these validated instruments should be used in conjunction with sound modifications in clinical settings that include patients, families, and nursing staff.

Future qualitative and quantitative research studies should be developed to test the effect of ambient therapy in surgical waiting rooms and phase 2 recovery environments. Additionally, the use of music and sound alteration techniques should include trials with select nursing staff. Using an ambient sound environment in staff lounges may mitigate the stress that operating room nurses experience. Compassion fatigue is a known consequence for personnel working in very high–stress environments, such as trauma centers. Trials using ambient nature sounds and accompanying musical compositions instead of the typical break-room milieu may provide valuable data that may affect future designs in health care support spaces.

Summary

The primary purpose of this article is to stimulate scientific inquiry into alternative means of reducing stress, pain, and anxiety for patients, visitors, and staff. The extent and potential value of these concepts may appreciably augment current therapies for patients. The influence of psychoacoustics and control of ambient noise floor for visitors and nursing staff has not been explored. Understanding the influence, or lack of influence, of these measures will substantiate the evidence needed for future designs in health care facilities.

References

[1] Young-Mason J. Music therapy: a healing art. Clin Nurse Spec 2002;16(3):153–4.

[2] Watkins G. Music therapy: proposed physiological mechanisms and clinical implications. Clin Nurse Spec 1997;11(2):43–50.

[3] Migneault B, Girard F, Albert C, et al. The effect of music on the neurohormonal stress response to surgery under general anesthesia. Anesth Analg 2004; 98:527–32.

[4] Ganidagli S, Cengiz M, Yanik M, et al. The effect of music on preoperative sedation and the bispectral index. Anesth Analg 2005;101:103–6.

[5] Wang S, Kulkarni L, Dolev J, et al. Music and pre-operative anxiety: a randomized, controlled study. Anesth Analg 2002;94:1489–94.

[6] Nilsson U, Rawal N, Unosson M. A comparison of intra-operative exposure to music—a controlled trial of the effects on post-operative pain. Anesthesia 2003;58(7):699–703.

[7] Good M. The lived experience of listening to music while recovering from surgery. J Holist Nurs 2000; 18(4):378–90.

[8] Diette GB, Lechtzin N, Haponik E, et al. Distraction therapy with nature sights and sounds reduces pain during flexible bronchoscopy: a complimentary approach to routine analgesia. Chest 2003;123:941–8.

[9] Stevens K. Patient's perceptions of music during surgery. J Adv Nurs 1990;15(9):1045–51.

[10] Palakanis KC, DeNobile JW, Sweeney WB, et al. Effect of music therapy on state anxiety in patients undergoing flexible sigmoidoscopy. Dis Colon Rectum 1994;37(5):478–81.

[11] Mok E, Wong KY. Effects of music on patient anxiety. AORN J 2003;77(2):396–410.

[12] Good M, Anderson GC, Stanton-Hicks M, et al. Relaxation and music reduce pain after gynecologic surgery. Pain Manag Nurs 2002;3(2):61–70.

[13] Frumpkin H. Healthy places: exploring the evidence. Am J Public Health 2003;93(9):1451–6.

ELSEVIER
SAUNDERS

Perioperative Nursing Clinics 3 (2008) 95–99

PERIOPERATIVE
NURSING
CLINICS

Index

Note: Page numbers of article titles are in **boldface** type.

DATE DUE